FUNDAMENTALS OF CASE MANAGEMENT

Guidelines for Practicing Case Managers

FUNDAMENTALS OF CASE MANAGEMENT

Guidelines for Practicing Case Managers

Judith M. Siefker, MA, CRC, CDMS

Michael B. Garrett, MS, CCM

Anne Van Genderen, RN, BS, CDMS, CCM

Marci J. Weis, RN, MPH, CCM

PRO-West
Seattle, Washington

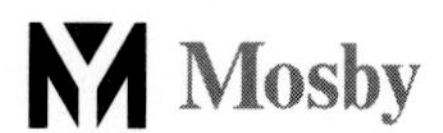

St. Louis Baltimore Boston Carlsbad Chicago Minneapolis New York Philadelphia Portland
London Milan Sydney Tokyo Toronto

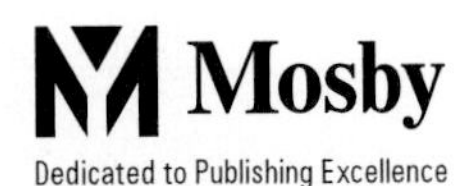

A Times Mirror
Company

Vice President and Publisher: Nancy L. Coon
Editor-in-Chief: Darlene Como
Editor: Yvonne Alexopoulos
Developmental Editor: Dana Knighten
Associate Developmental Editor: Kimberly A. Netterville
Project Manager: Patricia Tannian
Book Design Manager: Gail Morey Hudson
Cover Designer: Teresa Breckwoldt
Manufacturing Manager: Karen Lewis
Editing and Production: Book Production, Inc.

Printed in the United States of America
Composition by Book Production, Inc.
Printing/binding by R.R. Donnelley & Sons Company

Mosby–Year Book, Inc.
11830 Westline Industrial Drive
St. Louis, Missouri 63146

Library of Congress Cataloging in Publication Data

Fundamentals of case management : guidelines for practicing case
managers / Judith M. Siefker . . . [et al.].
p. cm.
Includes bibliographical references and index.
ISBN 0-8151-2498-8
1. Managed care plans (Medical care)—Management. 2. Medical
care—Utilization review. 3. Insurance, Health—Adjustment of
claims. 4. Insurance, Disability—Adjustment of claims.
I. Siefker, Judith M.
[DNLM: 1. Managed Care Programs—organization & administration.
2. Case Management—organization & administration. W 130.1 F981
1998]
RA413.F86 1998
362.1'04258'068—dc21
DNLM/DLC
for Library of Congress 97-16816
CIP

97 98 99 00 01 / 9 8 7 6 5 4 3 2 1

To all of the clients and patients
with whom we have had the honor to work.

PREFACE

Fundamentals of Case Management: Guidelines for Practicing Case Managers is geared toward case managers working for third-party payers and insurance carriers. It centers on case management as it is practiced in settings other than inpatient facilities, rehabilitation centers, and provider-based case management. Provider-based case managers can use this book to better understand payer-based case management.

This Book Provides the Following:

- *Training for new case managers who work in the insurance/third-party payer system.* Although this field is more than 20 years old, very few basic "how-to" books on this subject are available for case management trainees.
- *Guidelines for establishing and operating a case management program.* The book provides owners and managers with information on how to set up, manage, market, and improve case management firms and departments. Risk management and internal quality control are described for owners and managers to better manage the quality of case management services.
- *Information to improve the professional expertise of more experienced case managers.* Although this book is intended as basic instruction, it contains information on issues to which many case managers have not been exposed. Many of these subjects are included in Part IV, "Related Aspects of Case Management," especially vocational rehabilitation, disease management, the Americans with Disabilities Act, and cross-cultural issues.
- *Thought-provoking discussions of controversial issues.* This book is designed to encourage case managers to examine their values, ethics, and practices when performing their work. The authors present information on controversial issues objectively to avoid bias. At the same time, they encourage the reader to examine some of the pitfalls and subjects of debate that are of interest within the industry. These subjects include ethics, cross-cultural issues, who is qualified to be a case manager, and outcomes management.
- *A guide for non–case managers on how to work with case managers and what results to expect from case management.* This book is written with the lay person in mind, especially insurance adjusters and claims payers who purchase and utilize case management services. It helps dispel myths and misunderstandings about case management so that the purchasers of the service can use it more effectively.
- *An overall reference book on case management.* The purpose of this book is to serve as an easy and quick reference guide for fundamental information on case management. It provides basic information with cited references for more in-depth information.

This book was written as a joint effort by four professionals who have experience in case management, supervision of case managers, management of companies that provide case management services, utilization review, and vocational rehabilitation counseling. Anne Van Genderen and Marci Weis are registered nurse case managers. Michael Garrett and Judith Siefker have experience in vocational rehabilitation counseling, clinical psychology, and case management programs.

CONTENTS

PART I

INTRODUCTION TO CASE MANAGEMENT, THE HEALTH CARE DELIVERY SYSTEM, AND INSURANCE

CHAPTER 1

CASE MANAGEMENT: HISTORY, OVERVIEW, CONCEPTS, AND MODELS

HISTORY OF CASE MANAGEMENT

Although the profession of **case management** is relatively young, there is still some controversy about exactly when and where it originated. Indeed, case management probably has been practiced ever since people started to assist each other with health-related and social problems. Liberty Mutual is often credited with having pioneered the concept of in-house case management/rehabilitation programs in insurance companies in 1943 as a cost-containment measure for workers' compensation.[1] This concept was expanded in 1966 by Insurance Company of North America (now CIGNA) when it started an in-house program incorporating vocational rehabilitation and case management that later became Intracorp.[2] Some view George Welch of CIGNA as the true father of modern case management.[3] The early in-house programs of Liberty Mutual and CIGNA provided many of the basic components that are now considered integral elements of case management.

It has been stated that "the number of case managers has risen from an estimated five to ten thousand in 1985 to a total of fifty to one hundred thousand today, and this explosive growth will undoubtedly continue."[4] Although this statistic covers the past 10 years, case management has been around much longer. Case management as part of the insurance industry or other third-party payer systems seems to have had two somewhat separate origins: the workers' compensation system and the accident and health insurance system.

In workers' compensation, case management may be provided to individuals who are not severely disabled or ill but who are, nevertheless, experiencing difficulties in returning to work. Case management in this arena may focus more on nonmedical issues, such as job modifications and transitional return-to-work programs, than on actual medical concerns. The role of the case manager often overlaps with the role of the vocational rehabilitation counselor in workers' compensation work. This area is addressed in greater detail in later chapters.

Case management also originated in response to movements toward controlling the spiraling costs of health care in accident and health insurance. One of the major cost drivers is advances in medical technology, resulting in seriously disabled or injured people living longer with expensive assistance. For example, as of the 1960s, people with spinal cord injuries are living longer; in the 1980s, advances in treatment of head injury resulted in an increasing population of individuals with severe disabilities who needed long-term care; in the

1990s the AIDS epidemic substantially increased health care costs because new drug treatments extended the life span of those who are human immunodeficiency virus (HIV) positive. Case management is viewed as a way to control costs associated with this new medical technology by ensuring appropriate usage.

To control the costs of accident and health insurance, case management developed evolutionarily beyond utilization review to become a part of the larger umbrella of services that comprise managed care. **Utilization review (UR)** embraces a constellation of services aimed at ensuring that medically necessary care is delivered in the most cost-effective setting and manner while maintaining **quality of care.** When quality of care is compromised to save money, not only is the patient put at risk but costs may actually increase if the condition becomes worse as a result of inadequate care.

UR services generally include the following:

- Precertification review for nonemergent admissions
- **Second surgical opinion (SSO)** to ensure the medical necessity of elective procedures
- **Continued stay review** to ensure that patients are discharged at the appropriate time
- **Retrospective review** to evaluate the medical necessity of admissions or care after services have been delivered
- Hospital **bill audit** to ensure the accuracy of billing and the applicability of service delivery to eligible coverage

The need for case management can be identified during the delivery of any of these UR services through the use of various screening procedures and criteria. Cases are often referred for case management as a stand-alone service as well as a component of a number of managed care techniques.

UR services were initiated in the late 1970s by employers and accident and health insurance carriers who were alarmed by the double digit rate of inflation for medical costs. These interventions were focused on cost containment, but they were perceived to be adversarial in nature by health care providers and, to some extent, by subscribers and clients. This is because of the mandatory nature of UR, which usually carries financial penalties for noncompliance. Case management, on the other hand, is viewed by clients and providers alike as more collaborative in nature and empowering for the client. It typically is voluntary and has no financial penalties. Case management may also have the added benefits of providing research and education for making informed choices and securing additional services and payments for patients and providers.

Companies providing UR services often have screening methods for identifying cases with potential to benefit from case management. These screening methods usually take a variety of factors into consideration, especially the age of the client, severity of the diagnosis, multiple diagnoses, and ability of the client/family to provide care and resources within the client's community. Often, the screening criteria contain a list of severe or catastrophic conditions that are routinely considered for case management referral. (See Appendix 1 for examples of case management screening criteria.) These conditions are usually identified during precertification review and referred immediately for case management.

Workers' compensation referrals to case management are sometimes identified through routine UR services, but UR tends to be less widely used in workers' compensation insurance. More commonly, insurance adjusters at workers' compensation carriers will identify claims with potential to benefit from case management. The red flags that generally trigger referrals are as follows:

- Catastrophic injuries
- Use of extensive health care services for an extended period
- Multiple injuries or repeated injuries to the same part of the body
- Excessive time off from work
- Client seems to be getting worse rather than better
- Excessive use of prescription drugs
- Frequently changing physicians
- Presence of unrelated conditions that appear to be affecting the industrial injury or disease

The goals for workers' compensation referrals are to (1) resolve the medical issues, (2) empower the client to make informed choices, (3) return the client to work or assess the client's ability to return to work, or (4) develop a **vocational rehabilitation plan** that will assist the client in returning to work or becoming employable.

Case management became part of government entitlement programs in 1971, when the US Department of Health, Education and Welfare funded a case management demonstration project to integrate social and health services for clients.[5] Case management is now used routinely in many governmental programs, such as Medicaid, Medicare, the Department of Veterans Affairs, and the Civilian Health and Medical Program of the Uniformed Services (CHAMPUS).

Case management is practiced in many settings and does not necessarily involve only the management of medical services. Many case managers work within inpatient settings or as part of other types of service delivery programs. Although this book recognizes the varied roles of these case managers, *its focus is on insurer-funded or payer-funded case management, not consumer-funded or provider-based services.* The service described here is often referred to as *independent case management* because the case manager is not directly affiliated with insurance companies, although the payer is the main purchaser of the case management services described in this book.

A DEFINITION OF CASE MANAGEMENT

In 1990 the National Association of Rehabilitation Professionals in the Private Sector (NARPPS) proposed that "Medical Case Management is defined as the process of assessing, planning, coordinating, monitoring and evaluation of the services required to respond to an individual's healthcare needs to attain the goals of quality and cost effective care."[6] In 1993 the Commission for Case Manager Certification put forth its definition of case management, which was based on earlier definitions from Case Management Society of America (CMSA): "Case management is a collaborative process which assesses, plans, implements, coordinates, monitors, and evaluates the options and services required to meet an individual's health needs, using communication and available resources to promote quality, cost-effective outcomes."[7] In 1995, CMSA indicated that "the basic concept of case management involves the timely coordination of quality healthcare services to meet an individual's specific healthcare needs in a cost-effective manner."[8] Despite the fact that case management, health care reform, and managed care evolved rapidly in the 5 years that elapsed during the formulation of these three definitions, the essential goals of case management remain the same: coordination of quality health care services in a cost-effective manner.

All of these definitions focus on addressing health care needs, but case management is actually the coordination of a much broader range of services that deal with many other human needs that may or may not have a direct impact on health and medical issues. Some of these needs are vocational rehabilitation, social services directed at personal and family issues, and counseling services that do not require the intervention of medical model-based treatment. Specific examples of services that may fall outside the health care delivery system that case managers might coordinate are return-to-work programs, vocational counseling, financial counseling, support groups for families, Big Brother/Big Sister programs, Meals-on-Wheels, counseling for victims of domestic violence, and parenting classes. Although these services may not be part of the health care delivery system, they may affect the outcome of the case in respect to the insurance claim and may have indirect effects on the physical well-being of the client.

The NARPPS definition and the CMSA definition indicate that *medical case management* formerly was the term applied to the services that are now referred to as *case management.* The change in the terminology that designates the profession reflects the recognition that case management now has a broader focus than health care delivery and medical issues. Thus case management deals with the whole person, not just health-related issues.

This expanded model of case management to address the needs of the whole person is more effective in addressing the traditional twin goals of quality and cost-effective health care. To maximize medical independence and control costs, it is often necessary to go outside the traditional health care system to address family needs, cultural issues, emotional problems, financial concerns, work-related problems, and other nonmedical issues that may impede progress. For example, a woman who is going through a high-risk pregnancy may also have a history of domestic violence with her husband. Although the domestic violence would not be directly related to the medical risks of the pregnancy, physical beatings could certainly have an impact on the outcome of the pregnancy. If the insurance policy did not include counseling or mental health benefits, the case manager might seek help for the woman through a local domestic violence program that provides services at no charge.

Most human services professions now recognize the value of a holistic approach such as this because it encompasses the concept of patient or client empowerment. To achieve maximum success, the client and all other parties involved must work together to achieve common goals. The active participation of the client is an essential ingredient in achieving positive case outcomes of all types.

One useful way to picture the roles of the various players in the case management process is to use the analogy of a wheel. The client is the hub, and the other parties are the spokes. These individuals include physicians, other medical providers, treatment facilities, case managers, and insurance or third-party payer personnel. By functioning as the hub, the client is empowered by communication with the spokes to make informed choices and to pursue an organized and goal-directed plan of care that involves the active participation of the client in the recovery or **disease management** process. Together, the hub and the spokes hold the rim of the wheel together, which enables the whole unit to make progress toward designated goals.

Using a holistic approach requires the case manager to be a generalist with a wide variety of knowledge and skills. Not only must the case manager have medical expertise, but he or she also needs counseling skills, a wide knowledge of community resources, possible vocational expertise, mental health expertise, sensitivity to multicultural issues, proficiency in doing research, finesse in working with individuals with widely differing viewpoints, and a high level of ingenuity and problem-solving ability. Acquiring and maintaining all these different types of expertise make case management an extremely challenging but interesting occupation.

WHAT CASE MANAGEMENT IS NOT

Case management is not UR, although it may contain elements of this service. Case management may prevent unnecessary admissions and procedures and may reduce the number of inpatient days, but these are not primary functions. UR functions are aimed mainly at controlling costs. Although cost containment is an element in case management, its primary focus is on coordination of services to ensure quality of care and optimal outcomes.

Case management is also not the same as managed care, although it may be a component of managed care. It has been said that **managed care** is "a system of healthcare delivery aimed at managing the cost and quality of access to healthcare."[9]

SERVICES INCLUDED IN CASE MANAGEMENT

Case management generally begins with a thorough assessment, followed by plan development that takes into consideration the options available to satisfy the care needs of the patient and the benefit plan. The case manager must look at all relevant aspects of the case to determine the needs of the client and possible options for addressing them. The assessment involves obtaining information from many sources, including the client and family, attending physician, other medical providers, treatment facilities, vendors of medical supplies and equipment, employers, social service agencies, and others. Sometimes, the assessment involves research of the medical literature to obtain information that is not readily available from other sources.

Often, the assessment phase is the most crucial step in the process of case management. Without accurate and complete information, it is not possible to provide case management services that are truly beneficial and empowering to the client, that adhere to the benefit structure, and that provide cost containment for the insurer. Incomplete information can lead to oversights that compromise quality of care, are not helpful to the client in making informed choices, and lead to unnecessary expenditures.

The other extreme is to be avoided also. Sometimes, case managers in their zeal for thoroughness overassess and overevaluate, tracking down every possible factor that might influence the case. This can become a cost driver rather than a cost-containment service in case management. A compromise needs to be struck to obtain only the information needed to develop an adequate plan for case management.

Following a thorough assessment, the case manager develops a plan for how the case will be worked. A major component of this process is education and empowerment of the client to make informed choices in which he or she will feel invested and able to actively participate. To accomplish this, the case manager needs to have good counseling and communication skills. In developing the plan with the client, the case manager may assign some of the activities to be performed to the client to complete. Additional information has to be obtained, and options have to be explored. The client may require additional examinations and services, and ultimate outcome goals have to be determined.

To maximize the effectiveness of the plan, it is usually written in a step-by-step manner and is reviewed periodically to ensure that it is still valid and current. The written plan may be shared with the client/family, attending physician, medical facility, and others to ensure proper coordination.

Working the case involves coordination and referral related to the many diverse elements of the case, especially the exploration of benefits exceptions. The client undergoes necessary care and treatment, which is arranged, researched, and coordinated by the client and case manager in collaboration with the attending physician. As the case is worked, the case manager monitors outcomes and progress on an ongoing basis and takes corrective action as necessary as factors on the case change. The client is also empowered to take an active role in monitoring progress and initiating corrective action. Ongoing communication (both written and verbal) takes place with relevant parties (e.g., client, physician) to ensure compliance with the plan and resolution of conflicts or disputes.

The elements of the case management process (assessing, planning, coordinating, making referrals, monitoring medical progress, filing of proper forms for certain jurisdictions, monitoring outcomes and effectiveness of the plan, determining case closure, and transfer of the case at time of closure) do not take place in discrete steps that follow one another. To some extent, all of these elements occur simultaneously, although there may be more emphasis on one or more during certain phases of the case management process.

SUGGESTED READINGS

Bower KA: *Case management by nurses,* Washington, DC, 1991, American Nurses Association.

Cohen EL, Cesta TG: *Nursing case management: from concept to evaluation,* ed 2, St. Louis, 1993, Mosby.

Donovan MR, Matson TA: *Outpatient case management: strategies for a new reality,* Chicago, 1994, American Hospital Publishing.

Gerson V: George T. Welch: the father of modern case management, *Case Manager,* pp 71-75, Sept-Oct 1996.

Merrill JC: Defining case management, *Business and Health* 3(5-9):5-9, 1985.

Mullahy CM: *The case manager's handbook,* Gaithersburg, Md, 1995, Aspen.

Powell SK: *Nursing case management,* Philadelphia, 1996, Lippincott-Raven.

Romaine DS: Case management challenges, present and future, *Continuing Care* 14(1):24-31, 1995.

St. Coeur M, editor: *Case management practice guidelines,* St. Louis, 1996, Mosby.

Satinsky MA: *An executive guide to case management strategies,* Chicago, 1995, American Hospital Publishing.

Strassner LF: The ABCs of case management: a review of the basics, *Nurs Case Management* 1(1):22-30, 1996.

References are found at the end of the book.

CHAPTER 2
THE ROLE AND QUALIFICATIONS OF THE CASE MANAGER

A DAY IN THE LIFE OF A CASE MANAGER

Cynthia B. has elected to work at home today because she will be doing some paperwork and some phone work that can be done more efficiently without the distractions she encounters at the office. Later in the day, she will drop by the office to pick up her mail when she is on her way home from an appointment.

The company Cynthia works for gives her the option of working either in the office or at home. She has set up workstations both at home and in the office. The company provides her with a personal computer at home that is linked to the network of personal computers at the office via modem and fax. Some of the case managers employed at the same company as Cynthia rarely visit the office because they serve outlying areas that are a considerable distance from the office. It is more cost efficient for the company to equip them with what they need to set up home offices than to establish a formal office for each person.

Cynthia's day begins with the writing of two progress reports that she faxes to her supervisor. Her supervisor faxes them back to her by late afternoon; she makes a few corrections and then prints and mails them to the referral source. These progress reports describe what has happened recently on two catastrophic cases that will require long-term case management. Both of these cases involve intensive work that requires in-person visits to the client and various medical providers.

Next, Cynthia makes a number of phone calls on cases that are being managed telephonically. Mr. Y., a client who received multiple injuries in a motor vehicle crash, is scheduled to leave an inpatient facility within 24 hours and requires discharge planning. He will be returning to his home, but because his wife is frail and elderly and no other family members are in the area, he will need a visiting nurse, hourly home care, and durable medical equipment on a temporary basis.

Hourly home care is not covered by Mr. Y.'s medical insurance plan, which is designed to supplement Medicare, as Mr. Y. is retired. However, if Mr. Y. does not have hourly home care, it is likely that he will have to remain in the hospital for as much as a week longer because it will not be safe to discharge him to his home and the care of his wife. Cynthia anticipated this issue several days ago and contacted the **carrier** to discuss the advantages of making a benefits exception. Cynthia was able to persuade the carrier to make this benefits exception because she had researched the costs of the additional hospital days versus the costs of the needed additional services.

Cynthia contacts a home health agency that will supply a visiting nurse and hourly home care for 8 hours a day to assist with dressing changes, bathing, and a home exercise program. Cynthia also arranges for the rental of a hospital bed, a walker, and a wheelchair. Because Mr. Y. will be needing this equipment for a month, Cynthia requests a monthly rate. Although this rate is reasonable, she is able to negotiate an additional discount because the payer is a regular customer of the **durable medical equipment (DME)** supplier. The monthly rental rate is less costly than purchasing the equipment.

Arrangements are also made for a cab company with wheelchair vans to transport Mr. Y. from the hospital to his home. When all the arrangements have been made, Cynthia places calls to the hospital **discharge planner,** the payer, and Mr. Y.'s spouse to update them and address any unresolved issues.

Although Cynthia has never actually met Mr. Y. and his wife, she is aware of their needs because he was identified as having potential to benefit from case management through UR screening. This case was initially referred for continued stay review through a program mandated by the insurance carrier of a major employer for its retirees. Because of the age of the client and the number and severity of his injuries, the case met the screens established by the utilization review provider to identify cases with potential for case management. On receiving approval from the carrier to proceed with case management, Cynthia contacted Mr. Y.'s attending physician, his wife, and the hospital discharge planner to discuss his case. His needs were identified, and a date and place for discharge were established. Cynthia developed a basic written plan of services that would be needed to accomplish Mr. Y.'s safe discharge to home on the targeted date.

That afternoon, Cynthia meets with another client, Ms. S., and her attending physician at the physician's office. The purpose of this visit is to discuss possible reasons Ms. S. continues to have severe back pain that prevents her from returning to work. This three-way discussion reveals that Ms. S. is suffering from depression and is not sleeping well. The attending physician decides to start Ms. S. on a course of antidepressants. The attending physician also recommends referring Ms. S. for counseling. (Cynthia knows she must discuss this with the carrier before arranging the referral because benefits are limited for mental health services; she puts this task on her "to-do" list.)

Ms. S. makes an appointment for a check-back in 3 weeks. Cynthia makes a note to herself to recontact the physician by phone following this appointment for an update on Ms. S.'s progress and to discuss other alternatives if necessary.

While picking up her mail at the office, Cynthia looks up some medical information in one of the reference books available at the office. When Cynthia's supervisor sees her working at her desk, she asks Cynthia about a difficult case that has been of concern to both of them. Together, Cynthia and her supervisor review the case briefly, and Cynthia writes a new action plan in the case notes that she keeps in the file.

ESSENTIAL ELEMENTS OF THE CASE MANAGER'S ROLE

The example given illustrates that the essential elements of the case manager's role are communication, education, professional assessment of client/family needs, researching and making cost-effective recommendations, making recommendations for benefits exceptions when appropriate, review and coordination/monitoring of care and treatment plans, advocacy/mediation, and coordination with payer.[10]

Personnel in the insurance industry often find that the services of case management overlap, to some extent, with their role in adjusting the **claim.** Both roles are part of a philosophical trend toward controlling insurance costs by containing medical expenditures. However, the role of the case manager extends far beyond ensuring that claims dollars spent on medical care are used in the most cost-effective manner. Although that may be an insurance carrier's ultimate aim for instituting a case management program, the focus is much broader than merely getting the most service for the least dollars and preventing overutilization and inappropriate utilization.

The expertise of the case manager serves as a source of specialized consultation for the claims **adjuster** and expands the knowledge base of the adjuster somewhat. The case manager uses his or her expertise to take a broader view of medical and related issues on the claim to assess needs and research alternatives to develop a plan that addresses the needs of both the payer and the client in ways that benefit both.

Let us examine some of the individual functions of the case manager. Although these activities are described as being discrete functions, most of them tend to take place simultaneously rather than sequentially. For example, most of the assessment activities may take place early in the case, but assessment is also an ongoing process to determine if desired results are being obtained as a result of the treatment plan and other case management services.

The *CCM Certification Guide* identifies six essential activities of the case manager: (1) assessment, (2) planning, (3) implementation, (4) coordination, (5) monitoring, and (6) evaluation.[11] Adhering to the standards of practice for case management is crucial for the growth of the profession and the individual case manager's own competence and expertise.[12] The six essential activities of case management are addressed below along with some additional activities.

Assessment

Assessment is discussed at length in a later chapter because it plays such a pivotal role in case management. For case management to be effective, all relevant client/family needs must be identified and assessed. As well as medical expertise, this type of assessment also requires good counseling, interviewing, and observation skills. Needs assessment goes far beyond medical issues. It also encompasses financial, social, vocational, and other issues. The case manager has to be versatile enough to address these issues as well as pertinent medical ones. However, this does not mean that the case manager has to be an expert on all aspects of the case. It does mean that he or she needs to be able to access relevant information from other sources in the community, including physician advisors, other providers, community social service agencies, databases, and reference materials. Being a case manager is similar to being a librarian. It is not necessary to personally know all of the information, but merely to know how to access it.

Planning

Once the case manager has performed a needs assessment on the case, the next step is to make recommendations to address those needs. Often, the case manager must perform some research to determine what options are available and which ones will most effectively address the client's needs. This involves such activities as learning about the benefits that are available to the client under his or her **coverage,** negotiating with providers to address special needs or concerns, comparison shopping, and negotiating more favorable rates or service delivery packages. Once the needs and means for addressing them have been identified, they should be incorporated into a written plan that is action oriented, with specific time frames. An integral component of the planning process is the empowerment of the client/family to take part in researching options and making informed decisions.

Implementation

Implementation involves the execution of the case management plan to achieve the goals and also includes empowerment of the client/family to participate fully in the recovery program.

Coordination

Coordination is "the process of organizing, securing, integrating, and modifying the resources necessary to accomplish the goals set forth in the case management plan."[13] This is done on an ongoing basis for an extended period of time on some cases as part of the implementation of the case management plan. Sometimes, the case is closed after making the initial recommendations and initiation of the implementation process.

To implement some recommendations, considerable coordination is required to address multiple issues. The case manager is often the person designated to perform this leg work, although he or she may be assisted by the client, family members, hospital discharge planners, and others. Coordination of care may include linking the client to needed services, planning services, and identifying resources.

Monitoring

When case management benefits are limited, sometimes monitoring of care is not included. When monitoring of care is involved, the goal is to ensure that the treatment plan is safe and effective and is revised or altered when appropriate. If the case is a serious or catastrophic one, additional issues or concerns may present themselves frequently. It is the role of the case manager to address these ongoing problems in a timely and effective manner so that medical improvement continues with a minimum of setbacks. Involvement and empowerment of the client/family also are integral aspects of this phase of case management.

Evaluation

During the coordination and monitoring phases, the case manager is constantly communicating with the client/family, medical providers, and other significant players to determine whether the plan is being implemented properly and is achieving desired outcomes and goals. This evaluation process goes hand in hand with other case management activities because when desired goals and outcomes are not being achieved, the case manager must work constantly with others on the case to revise, implement, coordinate, and monitor new or revised plans.

Creativity and excellent problem-solving skills are essential to the performance of these activities as well as of those listed below. Case managers must be flexible in their thinking to identify options to address difficult and multifaceted problems.

The additional activities described below are also critical to successful case management, particularly empowerment of the client/family.

Communication

Communication takes place constantly during case management. One of the roles of the case manager is to facilitate communication between and among parties who ordinarily might not communicate directly or in an effective manner. Communication is made telephonically, in person, and in writing through correspondence, case notes, and reports. Because of the widespread use of computers, it is also made electronically through modem transfers and e-mail.

Communication is also essential to some of the other roles of the case manager, such as assessing client/family needs, coordinating care, and researching options. Although the different parties on the case (i.e., client, family, payer, medical providers) could all communicate with each other directly to achieve the same ends, mechanisms often are not in place for them to do so. Also they sometimes do not understand each other because of the use of terminology that means different things to different people and misconceptions about each other's roles. Often, the case manager translates the medical providers' technical jargon into layperson's terms for the medical providers and the client/family to ensure that they have the knowledge to make informed decisions.

Sometimes there is not enough time for adequate communication, and sometimes, resolution of certain issues requires in-person visits, which may be impossible if the parties who need to share information are located in different areas. Addressing some concerns may require a level of expertise that some of the parties do not have. At times, the parties may not know what the relevant issues are without the intervention of a third person acting as a facilitator.

Communication is essential to the successful performance of the other roles of the case manager. Options cannot be discussed, information cannot be obtained, and decisions cannot be made without effective communication. This role of communication facilitator distinguishes the case manager as an impartial advocate of the interests of all parties. It is also essential to the role of the case manager as educator.

Education

The case manager often has an educational role in working with all parties on the case. Essentially, the case manager is a knowledge and information broker. One role is educating the client on his or her medical and/or psychosocial condition, treatment options, and possible adverse effects so that the client can make informed choices or will cooperate with the recommended treatment plan. The case manager may also supply the physician and other health care providers with information that they may not be able to access easily. For example, without making a home visit, it may not be possible to know some of the conditions in a client's living situation that might impede medical progress. The case manager makes the home visit and problem-solves relevant issues with the medical providers, claims payer, and client/family.

There is also a caveat in educating the client/family. Sometimes, the attending physician has chosen not to share certain information with the client/family. The case manager must be cognizant of what the client knows about the medical situation and be willing to honor the attending physician's judgment in this. The goal of education is to empower the client and family in decision making.

Recommendations for Benefits Exceptions When Appropriate

Part of the process of making recommendations may include cost comparisons to suggest benefits exceptions to the carrier when the carrier is likely to save money in the long run. Careful research must be done when recommending benefits exceptions to ensure that the recommendations will truly result in cost savings and meet the approval of the health plan.

Advocacy and Mediation

The advocacy role is a tricky one because the professionals who become case managers traditionally think of themselves as client or patient advocates. In case management, advocacy is impartial, which means that the case manager advocates for all parties when it is appropriate to do so to achieve the dual goals of **cost containment** and appropriate quality of care. To use Freudian terms, the case manager is the "ego," which mediates between the "superego" and the "id" to achieve what is best for the client given the situation. At times, what the client wants either is not possible because the constraints of the benefit plan will place him or her at risk or is not feasible medically or socially. At other times, what the carrier wants is impossible to achieve without compromising quality of care. Providers want to earn a reasonable profit but are willing to give volume discounts to regular customers if the case manager advocates for the client and the carrier. Thus the case manager mediates and advocates among all parties to reach mutually agreeable decisions that will address the needs and constraints of all parties. The goal for case management is "everyone wins."[14]

Coordination with Payer

Coordination with the payer is obviously a component of most of the functions mentioned, but it deserves individual treatment because it is essential to case management. The payer funds the services of a case manager to obtain information about the claim, be educated or informed regarding pertinent issues, have the case managed in a cost-effective manner, obtain the opinions of an impartial professional, monitor quality of care, be apprised of the advantages of benefits exceptions, obtain information regarding **medical reserving,** and facilitate communication among all parties.

The reader is referred to CMSA's *Standards of Practice for Case Management* for additional information on the elements of the case manager's role and the activities of case management.[15]

QUALIFICATIONS REQUIRED OF A CASE MANAGER

Who is qualified to be a case manager has been a subject of discussion for a number of years but, as of this writing, remains somewhat murky. Also, some individuals and groups do not believe that case management is truly a separate profession because it has not yet developed a distinct body of knowledge.

The Commission for Case Manager Certification (CCMC), which awards the CCM (Certified Case Manager) designation to eligible case managers, has changed its criteria for eligibility somewhat since its inception in the early 1990s.[16] As of this writing, the minimum educational requirement is completion of a "post-secondary program in a field that promotes the physical, psychosocial, or vocational well-being of the persons being served. In addition, the license or certificate awarded upon completion of the educational program MUST have been obtained by the applicant's having passed an examination in his/her area of specialization."[17]

Acceptable employment experience is also a major focus for credentialing. All applicants must present verification of one of three categories of acceptable experience[18]:

Category 1	12 months of acceptable full-time employment or its equivalent under the supervision of a CCM for the 12 months.
Category 2	24 months of acceptable full-time employment or its equivalent. Supervision by a CCM is not required under this category.
Category 3	12 months of acceptable full-time employment or its equivalent as a supervisor, supervising the activities of individuals who provide direct case management services.

The Case Management Society of America (CMSA) also is not specific regarding education, work experience, professional licensure, or certification.[19] Following is a list of its qualifications[20]:

1. Maintain current professional licensure or national certification in a health and human services profession or both.
2. Complete a baccalaureate or higher level educational program for health and human services personnel.
3. Complete specific training and a minimum of 24 months of experience with the health needs of the population served.
4. Demonstrate knowledge of health, social service, and funding sources.
5. Maintain continuing education appropriate to case management and professional licensure.
6. Work toward and maintain case management certification.

The National Association of Rehabilitation Professionals in the Private Sector (NARPPS) does not address specific qualifications in its 1990 Professional Performance Criteria for Medical Case Management.[21]

Some individuals involved in the controversy over who is qualified to be a case manager believe that case management should be provided only by registered nurses. Some also think that only RNs with bachelors degrees or graduate degrees are appropriate. Others posit that only individuals with the CCM designation should be able to call themselves case managers. There is also widespread support for other certification, such as Certified Disability Management Specialist (CDMS) and Certified Rehabilitation Registered Nurse (CRRN).[22]

The reality is that many professionals who are not RNs and not CCMs and are not eligible for the CCM examination are working as case managers. Levels of competency vary, but as in most professions, this may not be in direct proportion to the number, levels, or types of credentials.

As mentioned in Chapter 1, case management is construed to be much broader than merely addressing medical issues. Therefore, although some cases are better managed by RN case managers or others with specific medical training, other cases call for professionals from other disciplines that are more oriented toward, for example, rehabilitation, vocational counseling, or social work.[23] Similarly, nurse case managers also have varying levels of expertise that range from extreme specialization (for example, high-risk pregnancies, AIDS/HIV) to generalists. Some cases are best served by generalists because a number of diagnoses and body systems are involved. Other cases benefit from the best specialist nurse case managers.

Essentially, most case managers function as generalists. They must know how to do many things, especially how to access many different types of information. RNs need to have clinical experience in a wide variety of areas because they are working with the whole person, not just a medical condition. Increasingly, however, companies providing case management services are offering case managers who are experts in a particular area of practice, such as head injury, psychiatric nursing, high-risk neonates, organ transplants, or orthopedic injuries.[24] Certainly, there are advantages to having someone with a high level of expertise in a specific condition functioning as a case manager. Less time will be spent on researching options, and significant issues are less likely to be overlooked. However, these specialists must also be able to be generalists in addressing medical issues outside their area of specialization and nonmedical needs/services.

Although it is beneficial to be able to advertise that one's company has highly specialized case managers for difficult, catastrophic cases, it is not advantageous to have only this type of case manager. Some cases involve multiple conditions and multiple issues that can be handled more effectively by a generalist who will not focus on one factor to the exclusion of other pertinent ones.

There are also advantages to having case managers who are not RNs if the essential issues on the case are nonmedical. For this reason, rehabilitation counselors and social workers often make excellent case managers. Some case managers with medical backgrounds may tend to focus only on medical issues and to overlook important social issues that may be impeding progress. Possible medical and nonmedical issues have to be balanced in selecting an appropriate case manager for a given case. If return to work is the central issue but the medical situation is complex, it may be helpful to have a nurse case manager and a vocational counselor working together as a team.[25] It has been observed that cross-training "is now essential for all who want careers in case management."[26]

The most significant factor is that all case managers must know and acknowledge the limitations of their professional expertise and always work within them. Adequate educational credentials form an indispensable base but are no substitute for experience. Continuing education must be an ongoing part of every case manager's career, but what is acquired from experience while performing casework is also essential. Case managers need to attend conferences, seminars, workshops, and classes on a regular basis and should also do professional reading to keep current in the rapidly changing and expanding field of medicine and related disciplines.

Because financial concerns are very important in many cases, a business background is also helpful. Case managers have to know how to make cost comparisons that involve many different factors. At all times, they have to be cognizant of the financial impact different options under consideration are likely to have.

A background in insurance concepts, especially claims administration and benefit plan design, is critical for case managers in successfully coordinating with insurance carriers. Carriers want to work with case managers who are knowledgeable about the insurance framework within which they must operate.

It is also critical for case managers to have a strong familiarity with the health care delivery system. Quick, proper accessing of necessary services, equipment, and supplies is likely to occur if the case manager knows the health care delivery system.

In addition to requiring knowledge of insurance and the health care delivery system and specific expertise for managing certain medical, vocational, financial, psychological, and social issues, case management also requires general competence in creativity, critical thinking, counseling and interviewing, negotiating, research skills, organizational ability, and problem solving. Flexibility in working with people who have many different points of view is also essential. Situations encountered in case management are often not black and white. There may be several options for achieving the same outcomes. Occasionally, after considerable research, it may still not be clear which option is the best for all parties concerned.

Emotional stability and strength of character also are important. Catastrophic cases often involve difficult decisions and tragic situations that test even the strongest of people. The ability to distance one's self and maintain objectivity when faced with these cases is extremely important. In general, these life skills tend to be ones that are not necessarily reflected in a person's education, certifications, job history, and examination scores. Case managers must remain cognizant of "care for the caregiver" issues to avoid burnout, promotion of client dependency, cynicism, overreacting to difficult situations, and so forth.

Last but not least, the case manager must have good organizational skills, including the ability to prioritize activities. Because speedy research and decision making often are essential in controlling costs while maintaining quality of care, the case manager must have the organizational skills and self-discipline to identify what activities have the highest priority and adhere to the priorities he or she has established.

SUGGESTED READINGS

Abramowski D, Arakaki A, Coyle J and others: NARPPS professional performance criteria for medical case management, *NARPPS J News* 5(6):111-115, 1990.

Case Management Society of America: *CMSA, Case Management Society of America, standards of practice,* Little Rock, Ark, 1995, Author.

Choppa AJ, Shafer K, Reid KM and others: Vocational rehabilitation counselors as case managers, *Case Manager,* pp 45-50, Sept-Oct 1996.

Commission for Case Manager Certification: *CCM certification guide, certified case manager,* Rolling Meadows, Ill, 1996, Author.

Engen CA: Certification: shining the light on excellence, *Continuing Care* 14(3):12-17, 1995.

Mullahy CM: *The case manager's handbook,* Gaithersburg, Md, 1995, Aspen.

St. Coeur M, editor: *Case management practice guidelines,* St. Louis, 1996, Mosby.

Smith DS: Standards of practice for case management: the importance of practice standards, *J Care Management* 1(3):6, 1995.

Specialized CM raises professional credibility, *Case Management Advisor* 5(8):108-112, 1994.

References are found at the end of the book.

CHAPTER 3
THE HEALTH CARE DELIVERY SYSTEM, MANAGED CARE, AND CASE MANAGEMENT

THE SERIOUSNESS OF ESCALATING HEALTH CARE COSTS

Health care costs as a percent of the gross national product (GNP) have gone from 5% in 1960 to 14% in 1992. This is much higher than any other country in the world. The United States and South Africa are the only two industrialized countries in the world that do not have some form of socialized medicine. There are 35 million uninsured people in the United States, representing 14% of the population. Because of rapidly escalating costs, health care purchasers, both the public and private sectors, have tried to control health care costs with a variety of strategies.

The total health care bill in the United States in 1992 was $838.5 billion, with projections of increases of 10% to 12% annually over the next few years. This greatly exceeds levels of inflation for the same years. The annual rates of health care insurance premiums in the 1980s increased 15% to 30% per year. For some policies and some groups of insureds, the rate of increase was even greater. The annual health care cost per employee went from $2000 in 1986 to $3500 in 1992, which represents a 75% increase in costs over 6 years or an average of 12.5% increase per year.

SOME FACTORS CAUSING STEEP RISES IN HEALTH CARE COSTS

Technology

There have been tremendous technologic advances in health care that have increased costs. These include organ transplants, expensive diagnostic equipment, new surgical procedures, and increasing ability to save and prolong the lives of catastrophically injured individuals who will need extensive care for the rest of their lives. Most of the costs of these advances in highly specialized treatment are reflected in the costs of health care plans.

Aging Population

With the aging of the baby boom generation, health care costs have increased, which will only be amplified as this generation moves into the Medicare program. This trend will continue well into the middle of the next century, and there will be another demographic blip as the current "Generation X" reaches old age.

Malpractice

The number of medical malpractice suits has grown, with increasingly high awards. This has resulted in increased malpractice premiums that indirectly get passed along to consumers or purchasers of health care. In addition, physicians have a tendency to practice "defensive medicine" to avoid malpractice suits.

Uninsured or Underinsured Individuals

Because about 14% of the population of the United States is uninsured, medical providers have many bad debts from individuals who cannot afford to pay for the care they receive. Consequently, the fees charged to payers tend to be inflated to cover these costs. Similarly, in some cases, Medicare and Medicaid fees are insufficient to cover true costs, and the discrepancy is **cost shifted** to the private sector.

Outpatient Care

With the intensification of inpatient cost containment, more health care procedures and treatments are being performed on an outpatient basis. However, the costs for these outpatient treatments and procedures are not necessarily less than they would have been if they were performed as inpatient treatments. In fact, sometimes providers charge more to perform these services on an outpatient basis because of the need for specialized equipment and personnel. Sometimes, higher charges are made for outpatient procedures to compensate the hospital for the costs of empty beds and other underused facilities.

Resources

Because of the limited supply of physicians, nurses, therapists, and other health care professionals, the salaries and benefit packages needed to attract and retain competent professionals have increased significantly in recent years. Since medicine is a worker-intensive field, increased salaries have a significant impact on overall costs. However, in some parts of the country, there is starting to be a surplus of medical personnel as a result of recent efforts toward health care reform.

Excess Capacity and Facilities

Hospital censuses tend to be low because fewer inpatient days are being authorized and more procedures are being performed on an outpatient basis. As mentioned above, cost shifting occurs to cover the cost of the overhead of empty beds and underused facilities. The closure of unprofitable facilities in some areas has increased costs because patients may have to be cared for in facilities that are considerable distances from their homes, thereby necessitating transportation costs and longer inpatient stays.

Drug and DME Costs

The cost of drugs and durable medical equipment (DME) has continued to rise during the past few years. This trend does not appear to be reversing.

Payment and Plan Design

Because most health care costs are paid by third-party payers, such as insurance companies or government agencies, the consumer has little incentive to reduce utilization. Plan provisions, such as copayments, have been included to correct this deficiency, but many plans do not cover some types of preventive treatment or evaluations that may save dollars through early detection and treatment.

Lack of Prevention

Traditionally, Western medicine has not focused on prevention, and there has been some resistance among insurers regarding prevention programs because it is often difficult to measure the effectiveness of such programs in real dollars. Despite this, however, the benefits of such preventive programs as well-baby care, routine mammograms, and routine physicals have been well documented.

MAJOR COMPONENTS OF HEALTH CARE FINANCING SYSTEMS

There are a number of different ways that health care is provided in the United States. Each system has both advantages and disadvantages. In recent years, various strategies have been developed to contain costs depending on the nature of the health care delivery system being used. The following examines the main systems for delivering health care and measures that are being used to control costs.

Fee-for-Service or Indemnity Plan

The traditional health care system out of which more recent ones have evolved is the **fee-for-service** or **indemnity** plan. The patient selects the provider, who determines the care required and sets the fees for services. In an unregulated fee-for-service system, there are no mechanisms to limit access to services or fees charged. The provider may bill the carrier directly for services, or the patient may submit billings for reimbursement. Most fee-for-service systems are now regulated in some ways to incorporate incentives for reduced consumption.

- Higher deductibles are often used to enlighten employees and subscribers about the costs of health care in order to encourage consumption of fewer services. Awareness of the cost of medical services is increased if the subscriber has to pay for a certain dollar amount of services out-of-pocket before insurance benefits begin to accrue.
- Copayments function in much the same way as higher deductibles to reduce utilization.
- Coinsurance limits or out-of-pocket maximums in benefit plans are similar to deductibles. They require the **subscriber** to pay a portion of health care costs up to a dollar limit.
- Sometimes, these financial incentives actually work against the goals of cost containment by discouraging preventive care. Consequently, some benefit plans offer free physicals, well-baby care, mammograms, and other services that are designed to encourage early diagnosis and treatment.

- Medical necessity language in benefit plans serves to more clearly define what services are covered.
- Emergency room treatment often involves an additional fee if the treatment does not result in an inpatient admission. This is designed to reduce costly emergency room treatment that could be done safely and effectively through physician office visits.
- Preadmission testing (PAT) is a requirement for patients to have certain diagnostic and other services performed on an outpatient basis.
- **Precertification**/continued stay review for certain types of inpatient admissions.
- Some plans have exclusions for court-ordered treatment, increased coverage for **home health care,** defined dollar coverage for transplants, increased coverage for **skilled nursing facilities** and other subacute facilities, and employee wellness and health promotion programs.

Despite some of these issues and regulatory mechanisms, many subscribers prefer this type of plan because they have broader choices of physicians or other medical providers.

Health Maintenance Organizations (HMOs)

An **HMO** is an organized system of health care delivery from designated health care providers available to a group of enrollees in a specific geographic area for a predetermined periodic payment. An HMO can provide a broader benefit coverage with emphasis on preventive care but within a specified network of providers that is closely controlled. The HMO Act of 1973 allowed for growth of this industry, and HMOs that agree to abide by the terms of the Act are given status as federally qualified HMOs. In return, these HMOs receive certain financial advantages. There are four general types of HMO:

1. *Staff model,* in which salaried physicians and HMO-owned facilities provide the care and services for the subscribers.
2. *Group model,* in which physician services are provided through multispecialty group practice that is independent of the HMO with which it contracts to provide physician's services. The HMO pays the multispecialty group at a negotiated per capita rate, which, in turn, usually pays the physicians a salary-plus-incentive for staying within certain parameters regarding costs and service delivery.
3. *Network model,* in which services are provided through the same mechanism as with the group model, except that the HMO contracts with more than one independent multispecialty group practice.
4. *Individual practice association (IPA),* in which services are provided by an association of individual physicians, including a mixture of solo and group practices, on a negotiated per capita rate, flat retainer fee, or negotiated fee-for-service basis.

HMOs generally focus on limiting access to specialized care by having the **primary care physician** function as a case manager who determines when the patient will be evaluated or treated by a specialist. In all four of the models described above, there may be financial incentives for the physicians for decreased or limited utilization. One of the main objections to HMOs is that this type of financial incentive compromises the quality of care that the patient receives. HMOs counter with the argument that this type of system encourages preventive care that reduces future illness, thereby controlling costs. In recent years, HMOs have also adopted incentives (usually in the form of copayments) for subscribers to decrease consumption of services.

Another objection to HMOs is that the patient has limitations on the choice of his or her physician. This is more problematic in some HMOs because of the small size of their staff or the small size of the IPA or group practice with which they contract. In larger HMOs, the patient is more apt to find a primary or specialty care physician to whom he or she can relate.

Preferred Provider Organizations (PPOs)

A **PPO** is a group of hospitals and physicians that contract with employers, insurance carriers, **third-party administrators (TPAs)**, and other groups to supply comprehensive medical care services to subscribers and accept negotiated fee schedules as payment-in-full for services rendered. There are six main methods of reimbursement for a PPO:

1. *Fee-for-service.* A traditional payment arrangement in which the financial risk is borne by payers, employers, and employees was the original form of reimbursement for providers.
2. *Discounted fee-for-service* arrangements in which the discount reduces the price per unit of service was the next step in financial reimbursement methodologies.
3. *Per diem arrangements.* The contracting hospitals agree to provide the room and board as well as the ancillary services for a specific amount per day, regardless of the number of services provided.
4. ***Diagnosis related groups (DRGs).*** This payment plan evolved from the Medicare system in which the payer contracts ro reimburse a specific amount of money based on a classification of illnesses, regardless of the **length of stay** or the number of services provided.
5. *Per discharged payment.* This strategy allows contracting hospitals to be reimbursed a set amount for each patient's hospital stay, regardless of diagnosis or length of stay.
6. *Per capita reimbursement.* This latest form of reimbursement involves providers' receiving a set amount per year per subscriber regardless of the amount of care provided or whether any care is provided at all.

A PPO is not an insurance carrier. It is a network of physicians and hospitals that provide discounts on services to plan sponsors in return for a volume of patients. One objection to this type of plan is that the plan sponsor receives the benefit of reduced payments per service, but cost savings may not be truly realized because the provider renders more services to make up for the losses on the discounts. Another concern is creative coding to disguise noncovered services or to gain higher fees to compensate for discounts.

Point of Service

A point of service plan is a combination of an HMO and a traditional indemnity or fee-for-service plan. The subscriber must decide at the time of service whether to go to HMO providers for service or to go outside the HMO network. If the subscriber goes to HMO providers, the care is usually reimbursed at 100%. However, if the subscriber chooses to go outside the HMO network, the care is reimbursed at a predetermined indemnity level less than 100%, such as 80%. This is similar to having a deductible or coinsurance provision.

Exclusive Provider Organization (EPO)

An EPO is a mixture of an HMO and a PPO. The EPO offers a network of physicians and hospitals to plan sponsors who, in return, require their subscribers to go to the EPO providers for their care to be covered by the plan. The EPO is *not* an insurance carrier, but rather it offers a network of providers to plan sponsors.

Integrated Delivery Systems

A new trend observed in health care is the emergence of **integrated delivery systems** (IDSs). This broad-based term covers diverse models involving strategic alliances among physicians, physician groups, hospitals, and other providers and practitioners. These new systems have been created in response to marketplace reforms and demands for better coordination across the spectrum of health care. The IDSs are now contracting with HMOs and directly with purchasers, sometimes on capitated contract arrangements.

There are a variety of ways in which an IDS can be created, and the rationale for the formation of the IDS depends on the governance and philosophy of the entity. Some IDSs want to preserve the autonomy of the providers within the system. Others want physicians to have the majority control of the organization, with little or no involvement from the local hospitals.

Ernst & Young consultants in Washington, D.C., have identified five major types of integrated delivery systems, including group practice without walls, individual practice association (IPA), integrated provider, joint venture, management service organization (MSO), medical foundation, and physician-hospital organization (PHO).[27] The type of IDS depends on several factors, such as function of the IDS, governance, philosophy and mission of the IDS, political climate of the health care environment, legislative and regulatory issues, source of the capitalization, and so forth. Regardless of the actual structure of the IDS, they are carving out new roles, and case managers will need to have a basic understanding of their processes and structures, since they may very well have patients who must access these systems. Also, case management firms may end up with an IDS as a client for case management services, and this will require an increased sophistication regarding these new entities.

Reasons for Development of IDSs

Competition. As the health care market has heated up with an increased focus on competition, providers have had to become more competitive with their services. An IDS is a way for providers to better market their services to purchasers.

Management and Marketing. More sophisticated management expertise and increased marketing efforts are needed in this new environment. The creation of an IDS can assist providers in having a vehicle through which they can professionally promote their services so they can obtain the contracts they desire.

Economies of Scale. There are new demands being placed on providers that make it extremely difficult for sole practitioners to continue to thrive. In particular, purchasers are requesting information systems and data report cards on performance, quality, access, and satisfaction, to name a few of these elements. This requires capitalization and collaboration with other providers, and an IDS may provide that vehicle.

Market Niche. Particularly with specialty providers (e.g., behavioral health), an IDS may be an opportune way in which to secure business. Large health plans may be very willing to contract out for specialty services even if they have been traditionally staff model oriented, especially if there is a well-organized system that can be used and is willing to share in the risk.

Reduced Hospitalizations. As health care has become presumably more efficient, there has been a concomitant reduction in the rate of hospitalizations. Obviously, hospitals see this as a threat to their survival, and new arrangements and collaborations are taking place. Forming an outpatient surgical clinic or other such service/product extensions is not enough to remain competitive. Hospitals see that they must reach beyond their walls to encompass the entire continuum of care into an attractive package for prospective buyers.

Organizational Issues that Confront an Emerging IDS

Governance. This has typically been the issue causing the most controversy in the beginning stages of an IDS. The role and control of physicians in relationship to hospitals are the key issues to be addressed in an IDS. Unfortunately, much attention has been paid to the issue of governance, and other issues may have been ignored or inadequately addressed.

Capitalization. Securing adequate capital for an emerging IDS is a real challenge, especially now that we are in the days of slim profit margins for health care as a whole. Inadequate capitalization may result in the failure of an IDS to survive.

Integration. Although an IDS wants to portray itself as an integration of health care, sometimes this is not the reality. This is especially difficult for hospitals who are involved in an IDS but who have not had to really work closely with ancillary service providers in delivering complete health care to consumers enrolled in a plan. Case management may evolve into the role of integrator of health care by assisting consumers through the ever more confusing maze of health care delivery systems.

Physician Compensation. Primary care physicians may be paid on a capitated basis in an IDS, which will result in a new perverse incentive to deliver less care in order to become more profitable. An IDS needs to address how it will check for this potential phenomenon.

Primary versus Specialty. The real battleground for the physician community is the role of primary care physicians and the role of specialists. Referral guidelines and practice standards are being developed to better delineate this situation, but it still remains a hotly debated issue. Case management may intervene by seeing that patients receive the care, treatment, and referrals necessary as defined by the plan or the IDS or both.

Regulation. If an IDS takes on capitated contracts, which is very likely, there is the issue of regulation and licensure by the state insurance commissioner. This is currently being debated by the National Association of Insurance Commissioners, and each state may address it differently.

Quality and Access Monitoring. As discussed above, monitoring the appropriate clinical quality and access to specialists will become increasingly important as new financial arrangements are negotiated. This will involve advanced information systems, provider profiling, development and implementation of critical pathways, development and implementation of improvement plans, feedback from case managers, consumer satisfaction, and other measures.

Risk Sharing. The issue of risk sharing will need to be addressed by an IDS, especially in light of capitated contracts. This implies sharing in both the gains and losses of the IDS. There are ethical and conflict of interest issues that arise with risk sharing for all providers in the IDS, including the case manager. (See Chapters 17 and 24 for further discussion.)

Network Development. The IDS will need to determine what kinds of providers and practitioners they want included in the IDS, so that targeted efforts can be made for these types of providers/practitioners. There need to be clear criteria for the inclusion and exclusion of providers/practitioners.

Competition. Many hospitals are forming systems to become more competitive. However, an IDS not only has other systems to compete against but also may compete with health plans with which it has contracts. In other words, an IDS may decide to offer its network to direct purchasers (e.g., self-funded employers), and this market segment is one for which health plans routinely compete. In the meantime, an IDS may have a contract with a health plan that is pursuing the same kind of direct contracting arrangements. This is happening so often that sales and marketing professionals have labeled it "competition." For one contract, the IDS may bid with a health plan with which it is competing on another contract. This kind of blended environment will be with us for some time to come. This also has implications for case management firms as they expand on their market base.

Major Implementation Issues in Managed Care

Credentialing and Recredentialing. The initial credentialing and then recredentialing of providers will need to be established. This will also apply to case managers who may need to hold licensure and also specialty certification (e.g., certified case manager) to be considered for inclusion in a health plan. Beyond the initial check on providers/practitioners, there will also need to be an ongoing assessment of the performance of the providers/practitioners included in the provider network to determine if improvement plans need to be developed in response to detected variations or deficiencies.

Utilization Management/Case Management/Quality Improvement Plans and Systems. A health plan will need to develop strategies for how it will address utilization managment, case management, and quality improvement for its network. Not only does this make good business sense for a health care organization entering into capitated contracts, but it is also being required of health plans pursuing accreditation from such organizations as the National Committee for Quality Assurance (NCQA) and the Joint Commission on the Accreditation of Healthcare Organizations (JCAHO). This may present business opportunities for independent case management and utilization management organizations in contracting for services with newly emerging health care systems.

Claims/Encounter Processing and Information Systems. As mentioned, purchasers and health plans are requiring more sophisticated information systems to produce data report cards and to monitor performance and outcomes. These systems tend to be very expensive and ever changing, so a health plan or an IDS will need to face the challenge of how to implement an information system within budgetary constraints.

Marketing/Sales. Health care organizations have not encountered the kinds of guerrilla marketing tactics other industries have had to face in the past. The predictions are that health care organizations, including the managed care industry and case management firms, will need to become very aggressive in their marketing efforts. Potential market segments will need to be defined, with appropriate distribution channels established.

Profitability/Survival. Depending on the charter of the organization (e.g., for profit or not-for-profit), the financial viability of the managed care organization will be extremely challenging, as there is increasing pressure to control costs while maintaining an acceptable level of quality and access. How the organization survives in this environment depends on how it meets the challenges outlined.

Comments

The purpose of this overview of managed care is to show not only that case management may find a viable new market segment with integrated delivery systems but also that to survive in this dynamic marketplace, case management firms will have to respond to many of the issues described above. Such issues as demonstrating quality, producing data report cards, credentialing, capitalization, and competition all apply to case management firms as a part of the larger health care delivery system evolution. Awareness of the issues is the first step in taking the necessary actions to succeed.

MORE ABOUT MANAGED CARE AND CASE MANAGEMENT

The difference between managed care and case management has been described as follows: "Managed care is a system of cost-containment programs; case management is a process."[28] Managed care is a major component in HMOs, PPOs, and EPOs. These health care delivery systems all feature major financial incentives for reducing utilization, streamlining services, and creating **sentinel effects** and **gatekeepers** who limit access to services. Managed care may also include such utilization review services as precertification, continued stay review, bill audits, concurrent review, and **retrospective review** and additional medical examinations, such as second surgical opinions, **independent medical examinations (IMEs)**, and **panel examinations.** It may also include what we have described as case management. Thus, case management is essentially a component of managed care.

One of the major differences between managed care and case management is that the former is generally applied to all cases and all subscribers, but the nature of case management is that it is only cost effective for a small percentage of cases. Managed care has cost benefits when applied to all **covered lives.** The 80/20 rule applies to case management. A rule of thumb in the insurance industry is that 20% of claims account for 80% of all the claims dollars that are paid out. It would seem logical that many of the cases that fall within the 80/20 rule would warrant the additional expenditure of case management services because there is potential for dollar savings as a result of case management. The purpose of case management in this context is to provide additional services that may not ordinarily be provided as part of managed care, with the hope of improved quality of care resulting in further cost containment.

SUGGESTED READINGS

Mullahy CM: *The case manager's handbook,* Gaithersburg, Md, 1995, Aspen.

Pies HE: Insurance and reimbursement: the ABC's of managed care, *Continuing Care* 12(4):25, 30, 1993.

Powell SK: *Nursing case management,* Philadelphia, 1996, Lippincott-Raven.

References are found at the end of the book.

CHAPTER 4

INSURANCE: GENERAL PRINCIPLES AND TERMINOLOGY

Insurance is a plan of risk management that for a price or premium offers the insured an opportunity to share the costs of possible economic loss through an entity called an insurer. Insurance is also a system whereby a large number of people or companies who are subject to the same type of loss pool a small portion of their resources so that when one suffers a loss, reimbursement for the loss will be made from the pooled resources. In other words, insurance is a method for sharing risk among a large number of people or other entities so that none of them will experience a financial hardship if one incurs a large loss.

Risk is a type of hazard that is insured against. Some common types of risks include fire, theft, auto accidents, and floods. Personal risks include the uncertainties surrounding loss of life, health, or income due to untimely death, illness, disability, unemployment, or old age. Property risks deal with direct or indirect losses to personal or real property due to fire, wind, accident, theft, and other hazards. Liability risks involve losses due to negligence resulting in bodily harm or property damage to others. Such damage could be caused by an injury on one's own property, by an automobile, by professional misconduct, or by errors and omissions.

Risk management is an organized plan of financial protection that persons or other entities devise to deal with hazards that they are likely to encounter in the course of their business or life in general. Some techniques for risk management include assessing the factors that may cause or contribute to the risk and taking steps to avoid or prevent whatever may cause the risk. Sometimes, a person or a company may personally assume the risk. For companies, this often takes the form of self-funding or the creation of a pool of money with which to pay claims. For individuals who elect not to have insurance coverage, this means paying for losses out-of-pocket or assuming the risk of having to take the consequences of not being able to pay losses (i.e., having to go through bankruptcy or having wages garnisheed).

Obtaining insurance through a carrier is one of the most frequently used options in risk management. This involves sharing of the risk with others. In the case of reinsurance, it may involve transferring the risk to another insurance carrier. **Reinsurance** or stop-loss is insurance for insurance companies or self-funded plans. If insurance is the preferred method of risk management, the first step in obtaining a policy is a risk assessment on the part of the insurance company. This occurs in everyday life when an auto liability carrier requests the driving record of a person who is seeking automobile insurance.

Underwriters are the insurance company personnel who decide what risks are insurable. Underwriting is basically a risk selection process that determines who and what are insurable. Because poor risks tend to adversely affect the insurance pool, thus increasing costs and premiums, underwriting is a very significant function in every insurance company.

For group insurance, the carrier may want to know such things as the age range of the population to be insured, their occupations, the hazards of their occupations, whether they live in rural or urban areas, and other factors. This information is obtained to assess the probability of loss and the costs that are likely to be associated with the loss.

Sometimes an insurance company will agree to write a policy for an insured but will not provide benefits under some circumstances or conditions. Certain services may also not be covered. These are called **exclusions.** There may also be limitations on the benefits or coverage for certain conditions and services. This is another way to control risk exposure.

The insurance company uses the risk assessment to determine the premium that will be charged to the individual or group for insurance. The amount of the premium is in direct proportion to the level of risk assigned. Companies or individuals often find various ways of reducing their risk to effect a proportional reduction in their premium. Case management and utilization management services are ways of reducing the risk of medical costs and, thus, controlling the costs of insurance premiums. For this reason, self-funded employers rather than carriers often incorporate case management programs into their health insurance or workers' compensation insurance plans to control medical costs and reduce premiums.

The *indemnity principle* holds that the owner of an insurance policy should be fairly compensated for a loss but not be allowed to profit by it. Thus, insurance only covers losses that create economic hardship and that have certain characteristics. The loss must be a significant one, and the loss must have a dollar figure attached to it. Vague types of losses, such as loss of pleasure or companionship, are problematic. The loss must result from an unexpected or unintended event, and the insurer must be capable of assuming the risk.

Premium rates are determined according to mathematical formulas as well as statistical and judgmental considerations. There are four major components that go into determining the amount of premium to be charged:

1. *Actual expenses of claims already incurred.* This cost is controlled partially by the quality of the claims adjusters and the cost-containment features of the insurance policy or plan.
2. *Retention charges or the insurance company's cost of doing business.* These include general administration and claims processing costs, state premium taxes, risk charges, and profit.
3. *Claim reserves.* These are funds held by insurers to account for costs in the period in which services are provided. Thus, there is a lag between the dates of services provided and the date the subscriber or provider is reimbursed for the covered services, so a reserve or claim liability needs to be established to account for this.
4. *Dividend margins.* These are intended to account for potential claim fluctuation, reduce the risk of understating the health care trend in premium calculation, and recoup losses from earlier plan years.

Premiums are calculated by *actuaries*, who are professionals who specialize in insurance mathematics. They also calculate rates, reserves, and dividends and produce statistical studies and reports through analysis, forecasting, and planning.

In the examination of the actual claims experience for a particular group, an insurance company or self-funded company carefully reviews the *loss ratio*. This is the ratio of actual claims experience to the premiums that have been paid. The targeted loss ratio will vary by insurance coverage and group size. If the loss ratio exceeds 100%, the insurance carrier has paid more in claims than it has collected in premiums. The loss ratio does not take into consideration expenses other than claims, such as administrative costs.

HEALTH CARE PURCHASERS

Those who purchase health care services are not generally individuals unless they are not eligible for a government program and cannot obtain coverage from an employer or a union. Purchasers of health care services are, typically, employers, government agencies, and union trusts. Employers may choose to purchase insurance to fund health care services from insurance carriers, or they may choose to be self-insured or self-funded. If they are self-funded, they may be part of a multiple employer trust (MET) or a multiple employer welfare association (MEWA).

Employers

Employers are the major purchasers of health care in the United States in the private sector. They purchase health care through two major plans: (1) workers' compensation, which is usually handled by a safety manager or a risk manager, and (2) health or medical insurance, which is usually handled by a benefits manager. Because of increasing health care costs, the chief financial officer has become involved in selection of the financing and delivery system selection.

Employers may use *brokers* (who typically are paid on a commission basis) or *consultants* (who are usually paid on an hourly or retainer basis) to assist in designing the benefit plan, financing the plan, selecting the health plan, and monitoring the financial performance. Employee benefits consultants are insurance professionals who, unlike brokers, do *not* work for a commission and do *not* usually sell insurance. Consultants specialize in the analysis and design of an employer's entire noncash compensation programs. Compensation to consultants is paid directly by the employer, usually on a fee-for-service basis.

Some large employers are choosing to be self-funded for various financial advantages (see discussion below).

Government Agencies

Government agencies involved in health care purchasing include the following federal and state programs.

Medicare. This program was instituted in 1966 as part of the Social Security Amendments of 1965. Medicare is administered by the Health Care Financing Administration

(HCFA). It was instituted initially to provide coverage for persons over 65 years of age, but in 1973, it was extended to cover persons with certain disabling conditions. In health insurance and long-term disability plans, case managers may consider coordinating the application process for Medicare coverage for those clients who have serious conditions that will last for 2 years or more. This could broaden the client's coverage and relieve the insurance plan of the financial risk of coverage.

Traditional Medicare covers inpatient (Part A) and outpatient (Part B) health care services, but it does *not* cover prescription medication. Enrollment in managed care plans, which typically include coverage for prescriptions, is increasing, however. Medicare supplements can be purchased to extend coverage and to pay for copayments and deductibles. There is much concern in this country about the growing Medicare population and associated costs because of the aging of the baby boomer generation.

Medicaid. Medicaid was instituted in 1965 under Title XIX of the Social Security Act. It is an entitlement program to provide medical assistance to a variety of low-income individuals who are eligible under certain programs, such as the Aid to Families with Dependent Children (AFDC) program or the Supplemental Security Income (SSI) program. The Omnibus Budget Reconciliation Act (OBRA 89) added pregnant women and children born after September 1, 1983, with incomes up to 133% of poverty level. Case managers may consider Medicaid coverage for certain pediatric and neonatal clients who, in addition to being covered by traditional conventional insurance, might be eligible for special coverage under Medicaid, for example, Early Periodic Screening and Diagnostic Testing (EPSDT).

Medicaid costs are shared by federal and state government, with the state responsible for the administration of the program based on guidelines issued by the HCFA. There are many concerns about Medicaid because of increasing enrollment and associated costs, yet eligibility and enrollment change monthly because of eligibility rules.

In 1981, Congress amended the Social Security Act to authorize Medicaid coverage of case management services under two provisions. (1) States were authorized to develop case management systems to direct patients to appropriate services. (2) States were authorized to furnish case management as a distinct service under home and community-based service waivers. In March 1994, it was noted that "40 states have started case management programs for Medicaid patients."[29] Case management has been focused particularly on Medicaid clients with chronic disabilities, since they tend to be high health care utilizers.

CHAMPUS. The Civilian Health and Medical Program of the Uniformed Services is administered by the Department of Defense. It serves the spouses and eligible dependents of armed forces personnel as well as retirees by providing coverage outside of the military health care system. CHAMPUS has had case management demonstration projects prove to be cost effective. Case management will be a key component in the new managed care support contracts CHAMPUS is awarding across the regions of the country to better manage their health care dollars.

Veterans Administration. The Veterans Administration covers eligible veterans for their health care needs and also provides a network of facilities and health care providers.

Indian Health Service. The Indian Health Service provides health care to Native Americans.

Public Health Service. The Public Health Service addresses a variety of health care needs in communities, such as providing immunizations and HIV testing.

Other Agencies. Some states have developed plans for the near poor who are not Medicaid eligible and are uninsured. There are also health plans for state, federal, and other government employees that are managed by governmental agencies.

Taft-Hartley Trusts

Taft-Hartley Trusts are created and funded through collective bargaining between participating labor organizations and employers for the health and welfare benefits of the members of the labor organization. They usually consist of more than one employer in a similar industry, such as construction. They determine the amounts to be contributed by the participating employers and the benefit levels to be provided. Some are also self-funded and must comply with the **Employee Retirement Income Security Act (ERISA)** as well as the Taft-Hartley Act. (See Regulation of Insurance Companies discussion for information on legislation related to ERISA and Taft-Hartley Trusts.) They are administered by joint labor-management boards of trustees with the assistance of professional service providers and may be governed by collective bargaining agreements.

Multiple Employer Trusts (MET) and Multiple Employer Welfare Associations (MEWA)

METs and MEWAs are usually groups of small employers that join together by nature of business or regional location to offer joint benefit plans to their employees. This kind of grouping helps small employers to obtain a better premium because of the size of the combined group. Some METs and MEWAs even become self-funded because of their size.

Individual Purchasers

Individual purchasers are people who obtain coverage through an individual policy. They must also pay copayments, deductibles, and excluded benefits; they also usually pay for part of the premium through an employer-sponsored plan.

Summary

It is important for the case manager to know who the health care purchaser is because there are different lines of authority in obtaining authorizations and benefits exceptions in each of these systems. Some of these systems also have other characteristics that the case manager must attend to in working the case.

SELF-INSURANCE/SELF-FUNDING

Sometimes companies self-insure for workers' compensation or medical insurance and sometimes for **long-term disability (LTD)** or short-term disability (STD). This involves the plan sponsor's setting aside money in a special fund from which certain types of claims will be paid. Usually only large companies have the financial resources to self-insure. Sometimes smaller companies that may all belong to the same industry join together to pool their resources to form METs and MEWAs in a self-funding arrangement.

Generally, self-funded plans are insured against exceptionally large losses by reinsurance or stop-loss. Reinsurance is a means of shifting part of the financial responsibility of one insurer (the self-funded employer) to another (the reinsurance carrier). An insurer places part of the risk with a reinsurance carrier and pays a premium for the amount of risk to be assumed by the reinsurance carrier. Reinsurance is actually insurance for insurers. The stop-loss is the trigger point at which the self-insured company or group's risk or liability ends and the reinsurance carrier's risk begins.

Stop-Loss

When a reinsurance carrier or stop-loss carrier is used by a self-funded employer, there are typically individual or aggregate (or both) stop-loss amounts or benchmarks set. An individual stop-loss amount is a dollar threshold for the claims costs for one subscriber/claimant at which the reinsurance policy is activated. An aggregate stop-loss amount is a dollar threshold for the claims costs for the entire covered population at which the reinsurance policy is activated.

It is essential that the case manager understand these thresholds in order to know who is at risk (i.e., the party responsible for paying the claims) when working the case. A case manager may need to coordinate and communicate with the reinsurance carrier when an individual stop-loss amount has been exceeded, for example. In fact, the reinsurance carrier may assume the role of authorizing and controlling case management activities once the individual or aggregate stop-loss amounts have been exceeded. The case manager and the firm need to be aware that the purchaser of the case management services can, indeed, become the reinsurance carrier in the middle of a case.

There may also be tiers of reinsurance carriers as claims costs increase. Thus, there may be one reinsurance carrier for an individual subscriber/claimant for claims costs from $100,000 to $199,000, another for claims ranging from $200,000 to $299,000, and so forth. An umbrella entity (such as the third-party administrator) may coordinate all of these reinsurance carriers, or the case manager may need to track claims costs and communicate with the responsible reinsurance carrier as the case progresses. Again, it is critical for the case manager and the firm to be aware of these aspects of a self-insured plan in order to obtain proper direction/authorization, receive prompt payment of case management services, assist in proper claims submission and payment, and communicate appropriately with all relevant parties.

Administration

Companies that self-fund may be self-administered, which means that they have in-house eligibility, administration, and claims operations. If a self-funded company does not want to be self-administered, it may contract with a third-party administrator (TPA), which is a company that specializes in claims administration and eligibility maintenance for self-insured programs. Another option for self-insured employers is to obtain an **administrative services only (ASO)** arrangement through a division of an insurance company.

Reasons for Self-Funding

Often the motive for companies to self-insure is to save money on insurance costs by directly controlling what claims are paid. In an effort to control costs, risk management is usually a prime area of focus for self-insured companies. Risk management can include many components but is often focused on occupational health and safety, managed care, and wellness programs. Other reasons for self-insuring include reduction or elimination of state premium taxes, reduction of general administration costs, reduction of insurer's profit margin, plan design flexibility, avoidance of state-mandated benefits (applies to health insurance only), cash flow, and better, more responsive service.

REGULATION OF HEALTH PLANS

Health plans and insurance carriers tend to be heavily regulated by both state and federal agencies. The reason for this is that serious problems ensue when insurance companies go into receivership or refuse to insure certain types of risks.[30] Insurance legislation varies considerably from state to state, but it generally mandates the amount and type of coverage and who must obtain insurance, as well as the financial stability of the insurance carrier. Most states have an insurance commissioner who regulates companies that write policies in their state and handles complaints. Companies that self-fund their medical benefit plans are exempted from state regulation by ERISA (see below).

Self-insurance for workers' compensation is often heavily regulated by state law to ensure that individuals who fall under the jurisdiction of self-insured companies receive the same coverage and benefits as those who are insured by insurance companies. Following are some federal laws regulating health plans and insurance.

ERISA of 1974

The Employee Retirement Income Security Act (ERISA) of 1974 governs self-funded health benefit plans that are exempted from state regulation, including state-mandated employee benefits plans and governance by the state insurance commissioner's office. This is called ERISA preemption. It also provides that employee benefit plans will *not* be deemed to be an insurance company or other insurer.

ERISA was intended to create a federal system for regulating self-funded employee benefit plans, including retirement and health insurance, in a uniform manner. ERISA claims are decided under federal jurisdiction by a judge, and jury trials are excluded. Punitive damages for extracontractual damages, such as "pain and suffering" and emotional distress, are also excluded. However, the plaintiff's attorney fees are recoverable.

One of the provisions of ERISA that is significant for case managers is that plan fiduciaries are personally liable to compensate the plan for losses resulting from a breach of fiduciary duty. However, case managers are not usually considered fiduciaries because they do not exercise authority over the management of the financial assets of an ERISA plan. Thus, because a case manager's role is usually advisory or consultative in nature, he or she usually cannot be sued for monetary damages under ERISA.

ERISA has a number of implications for case management:

- There is no recourse from the state insurance commissioner in the case of a dispute. Disputes are handled by administrative law judges (ALJs).
- Benefit packages may vary because they do not have to follow state-mandated plans.
- Damages for "pain and suffering" are not paid.
- The plan sponsor is in control under ERISA—not ERISA itself or the state insurance commissioner. This is beneficial because it allows for more flexibility for problem solving, but recourse may be limited.
- The plan sponsors have more latitude, but they may have the potential to discriminate under the Americans with Disabilities Act (ADA). For example, imposing a cap on benefits to AIDS patients may be considered discriminatory under ADA.
- Because regulations are limited, the case manager may be able to act as a resource to advise the plan sponsor on how to improve the benefit plan. However, the case manager should be cognizant of his or her limitations in this area. Case managers are not expected to function as employee benefits consultants or attorneys.
- Ability to make benefits exceptions may be hindered because all plan participants must be treated in the same manner.

COBRA of 1985

The Consolidated Omnibus Budget Reconciliation Act (COBRA) of 1985 is a federal budget measure that included a requirement for mandatory continuation of health benefits coverage for employees and their dependents who would otherwise lose their group health plan eligibility after terminating employment. COBRA requires employers to make health care plans available to former employees and qualifying family members. These plans are to be made available for a defined period of time. This legislation specifies rates, coverage, qualifying events, eligible individuals, notification requirements, and payment terms.

COBRA also has some implications for case managers:

- Because COBRA benefits are time limited, the case manager must take the termination date of the benefits into consideration when making long-range plans.
- The COBRA plan may cover a seamless transition to the next benefit plan (i.e., Medicare or Medicaid).

Taft-Hartley Trusts

The Taft-Hartley Act of 1948 allowed labor unions to form trusts to administer their benefits. These trusts are third-party beneficiaries of collective bargaining agreements that determine employer contributions and benefit levels. This type of trust is comprised of and administered by equal numbers of union and management representatives (with the assistance of third-party administrators) and may include a number of employers. Employer trustees are generally officers or managers of participating companies. The union trustees are generally officers or representatives of the participating labor organization.

In addition to health care benefits, Taft-Hartley plans may also offer employee group term life insurance and accidental death and dismemberment insurance. Health care benefits may range from catastrophic major medical coverage to paid-in-full plans. Some trusts (typically the largest ones) also allow their participants to choose among two or more coverage options.

Most trusts have experience with some form of managed care. The use of preferred provider organizations is commonplace. Utilization review and case management are common features in Taft-Hartley plans.

Because unionized workers often have short-term or part-time jobs with participating employers, the Taft-Hartley Act provides for portability of coverage within the trust and with other trusts.

Case management implications for Taft-Hartley trusts include the following:

- Union involvement causes these plans to tend to be more benevolent to patients than other types of plans.
- They may not be as objective as other plans in deciding who will get benefits exceptions (i.e., exceptions are often based on the individual's reputation with the deciding body).
- There may be **confidentiality** issues because the patients are often personally known to the members of the trust.
- Decision making may be a lengthy process because both labor and management are involved.
- Collective bargaining agreements sometimes get in the way.

HOW CASE MANAGERS WORK WITH INSURANCE COMPANIES AND OTHER HEALTH PLANS

Although many different functions take place in an insurance company, case managers are most likely to have contact with claims units and, to a much lesser extent, loss control. Claims units are composed of claims managers, claims supervisors, and adjusters. When a claim is made to an insurance company, it is usually assigned to an adjuster who is responsible for determining the validity of the claim and eligibility of the claimant/subscriber, assessing the dollar amount of costs that are likely to be associated with the claim (setting the reserve on workers' compensation cases), authorizing benefits that are paid (according to the fee schedule or usual and customary charges), and settling the claim. For some lines of insurance, different adjusters handle bodily injury and property damage claims. Some adjusters only handle medical claims.

Claims Adjusters

Claims adjusters work under claims supervisors. Adjusters may have to go to their supervisors for authorization of some types of payments on claims. This may be especially true if benefits exceptions are to be made or authorization is to be given for exclusions, limitations, or experimental medical procedures. Supervisors may also function as adjusters for some of the more complex or difficult claims. Sometimes, these complex claims may be handled by special units, and sometimes, it is necessary to go to the manager or superintendent of the claims unit for approval of certain expenditures.

Case Management Functioning

Some insurance companies have in-house case managers or private rehabilitation companies associated with them who provide case management. In many companies, these case managers provide the full line of case management services to claimants/subscribers. In other instances, the in-house case manager acts as a broker for case management services that are referred out to case management companies on a contractual basis. In this scenario, the in-house case manager would screen cases for ability to benefit from case management and would refer the case to an appropriate provider. The in-house case manager might also authorize services, review reports, go over billing, and function as a liaison between the claims personnel and the case manager.

In other insurance companies, the adjuster, claims supervisor, or claims manager would authorize case management services and make referrals to outside vendors. In working any cases referred by an insurance company, it is important for the case manager to know and understand the lines of authority in obtaining certain types of approvals and making decisions.

One important consideration is that every insurance company is different. Consequently, the case manager needs to learn how to work with each referral source on an individual basis. In working with a self-insured company, it is important for the case manager to know whether it is self-administered or has a TPA or ASO. If a TPA or ASO is being used, it may be necessary for the claims adjuster to contact the self-insured employer to obtain certain authorizations for case management and/or benefits exceptions. This creates an additional layer of authority, which often delays decision making. Sometimes, also, the TPA or ASO is reluctant to request special authorizations from the company that has hired it because it views the case manager's role as being in competition with its own role. This is often true when it comes to making referrals for case management.

Employee benefits consultants may also have some influence over whether case management is used in an insurance plan. Fig. 4-1 shows how an employee benefits consultant fits in the general scheme of things.

Generally speaking, how the case is worked will be affected by the type of referral source. Insurance companies are generally able to make authorizations without consulting the employers for which they write coverage. TPAs and ASOs usually have to obtain authorization from the company for which they work in order to refer claims for case management and make benefits exceptions. Referrals that come directly from self-insured companies are often extremely cost conscious. Because the client will be an employee or dependent of an employee, the self-insured company may also be very conscious of public relations issues and may be concerned about retaining a valuable staff member. There may be concerns

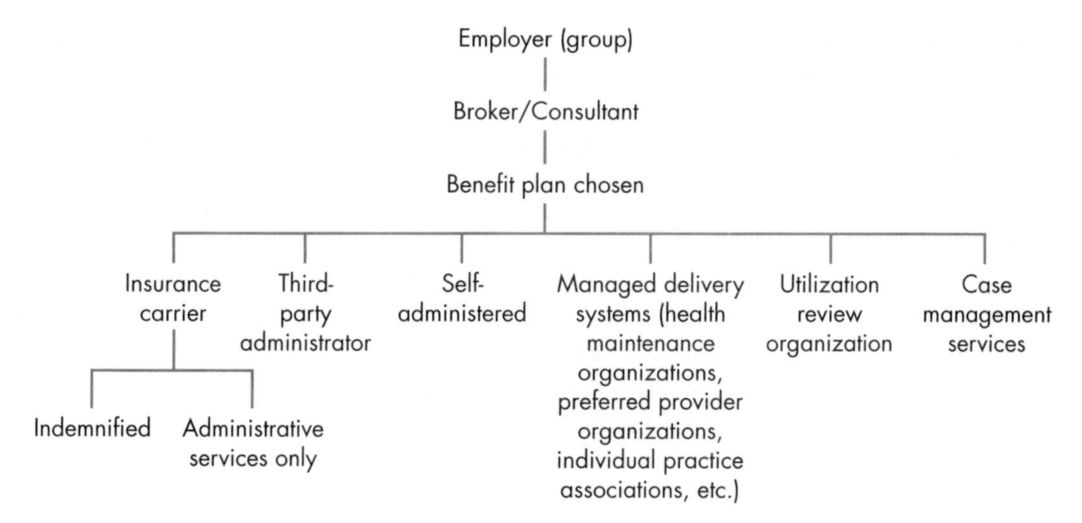

FIG. 4-1 Location of the employee benefits consultant in the health care reimbursement hierarchy.

that case management may convey to the employee that the company is interested in cost savings at the expense of the welfare of the patient.

Consequently, case management services must always be customized to address the needs and issues of the referral source. Working with government agencies that provide coverage may be especially complex because of public scrutiny and a plethora of rules and regulations.

HEALTH PLAN EXPECTATIONS AND OBJECTIONS TO CASE MANAGEMENT

The health plan may not always know exactly what it wants from case management, so the case manager may need to help to define the process and results that can be expected from case management. Therefore, it is the responsibility of the case manager to educate the insurance company on the benefits of case management in general and on specific cases. The insurance company needs to know what types of claims and what circumstances may warrant case management, the process of case management, and the outcomes that can reasonably be expected from case management.

One of the principal outcomes expected by insurance companies is *valid* cost savings that can be clearly documented. The insurance company also wants improved quality of care for their subscribers or patients through the work of knowledgeable and skilled case managers. Another common expectation is demonstrated improvement in employee or subscriber relations through the case management program. To address these needs, case management companies need to develop good techniques for measuring outcomes and reporting them. (This is discussed at length in later chapters.)

Conversely, customers are often concerned about incurring higher costs through case management as a result of recommendations for more expensive or extensive health care services or equipment. In this vein, concerns are often voiced that case managers will be too patient advocacy oriented to the detriment of sound **cost-benefit analysis.** Conversely, insurance companies are also concerned that case managers may be too aggressive, insurance oriented, and cost containment oriented to focus on maintaining quality of care for the patient. Sometimes, case managers are perceived as intimidating because the adjuster's medical knowledge is limited. Customers also fear overreferral of cases because of inadequate methods of screening claims that are likely to benefit from case management. Another frequently heard complaint is lack of comprehensive, timely, accurate data reports on the aggregate of claims as well as for individual cases.

All of these factors emphasize the fact that case managers and the firms they work for need to pay close attention to the expectations of the referral source in order to have a growing concern and to obtain repeat business.

SUGGESTED READINGS

Mullahy CM: *The case manager's handbook,* Gaithersburg, Md, 1995, Aspen.

Pies HE: Insurance and reimbursement: third party payment 101, *Continuing Care* 12(2):32-33, 1993.

Powell SK: *Nursing case management,* Philadelphia, 1996, Lippincott-Raven.

References are found at the end of the book.

CHAPTER 5

LINES OF INSURANCE COVERAGE

HOW HEALTH INSURANCE DIFFERS FROM PROPERTY AND CASUALTY INSURANCE

Property and casualty insurance protects against many different kinds of risks. Some of the most common types of property and casualty insurance that include case management services are workers' compensation, auto liability, auto no-fault, and commercial or general liability insurance. **Liability insurance** pays benefits for bodily injury and property damage that is incurred as a result of the errors, omissions, or negligence of a third party. To collect benefits from liability insurance, the **claimant** must prove that the insured was at fault or caused the bodily injury or property damage in some way.

Liability insurance generally has limits of coverage. This means that expenses or losses will only be compensated under certain specific circumstances and up to a specified dollar limit. The dollar limit usually has two provisions: an amount for each person involved and a total amount for the entire incident. It has been observed that "the coverage limits often determine whether [case management] services will be feasible. If limits are low and bodily injury is severe or catastrophic, it may be clear from the outset that the claim will exceed policy limits. If that is the case, there is usually no financial incentive to provide rehabilitation as a cost containment measure."[31]

No-fault is the opposite of liability insurance in the sense that it is not necessary to prove that an insured third party caused the damages. No-fault is just what it implies, an insurance system whereby bodily injury and property damages are paid regardless of who was responsible for the incident. Workers' compensation and **auto no-fault** are two types of no-fault insurance. In a no-fault system, lawsuits are not allowed except under certain circumstances, such as when there is a third party involved who is not normally included in the coverage. (For example, a machine was manufactured with a defect that ultimately resulted in the injury of an employee who worked for a company that purchased the machine for use in the course of doing business.) Health insurance can also be considered a type of no-fault insurance, although it is not considered a type of property and casualty insurance because it operates somewhat differently.

The other side of the insurance industry is called **accident and health insurance.** This terminology is somewhat misleading, as accident and health insurance does *not* include automobile accidents or other liability situations. Thus, accident and health insurance includes the following broad policies:

- Health/medical insurance
- Long-term disability (LTD)
- Accidental death and dismemberment

The type of accident and health coverage that is most likely to use case management services is health or medical insurance.

Health insurance only pays medically related expenses. It does not cover property losses, lost wages, and death benefits. It will cover a broad range of medical conditions and expenses except those associated with other insurance claims, such as workers' compensation and automobile insurance. Often, however, it will take over when the **benefits** limits from other types of insurance have been reached. For example, an auto insurance policy may only cover bodily injuries up to 3 years after injury or $10,000. When these limits are reached, the individual's health insurance may pay for additional medical expenses. Health insurance is explained more thoroughly in Chapter 3.

Property and casualty insurance usually will only pay claims for losses under certain circumstances. For example, workers' compensation only covers injuries occurring on the job. A commercial liability policy may cover a child who is injured on a playground at school. At times, who the responsible party is may not be clear, and the case will be controverted. For example, a worker may be injured in an automobile accident while on company business (workers' compensation insurance), but the person driving the other vehicle may be at fault (auto liability insurance) or the manufacturer of one of the vehicles may be responsible for a defective part that caused the accident (commercial liability). Box 5-1 illustrates a number of variables that differentiate property and casualty lines from accident and health insurance.

As you can see, the property and casualty market functions quite differently from the accident and health market. It is most important for the case manager to know what form of insurance is relevant when handling a referral for case management because it will affect goals, recommendations, and activities.

BOX 5-1

COMPARATIVE CHARACTERISTICS OF THE TWO MAIN AREAS OF THE INSURANCE INDUSTRY

PROPERTY AND CASUALTY	ACCIDENT AND HEALTH
Insuring for an event that may or may not happen	Insuring for relatively predictable events
"Risky business"	Relatively scientific and statistically based
Premiums collected annually	Premiums collected monthly or quarterly
Specific risk is insured that is clearly defined in the policy	Comparatively speaking, very little is excluded from this coverage
Claimant	Subscriber
Goal is to return to preloss status, nothing more	Goal is to indemnify, or make whole
"Should I pay this claim?"	"How fast can we pay this claim?"
Morbidity is the question (frequency of occurrences of events)	Mortality is the question (frequency of deaths in proportion to a population)

PROPERTY AND CASUALTY INSURANCE LINES

Workers' Compensation

Workers' compensation is insurance that provides for the payment of benefits for injuries or diseases incurred while functioning in an employment situation. The type, amount, and extent of such benefits will vary according to the laws of a given state.

Before the implementation of workers' compensation laws, which took place around the turn of the century, employees had to bring suits against their employers to collect benefits. Cases were rarely brought to suit because of the expense, and when they were, the onus was on the employee to prove negligence. When a suit was won by the employee, the employer could very well go bankrupt because of the size of the award. Because of legal delays and **appeals,** a considerable amount of time often would elapse between the injury and the award. During this time, the employee and his or her family would often suffer because no money was available for medical bills and income replacement. If the employee did not receive an award, there would be no financial compensation at all even though the injury might be quite extensive and debilitating.

Workers' compensation is, in essence, a no-fault type of coverage in which benefits are paid to the employee regardless of whether he or she, the employer, or someone else is responsible for the injury. However, workers' compensation laws hold the employer liable on the basis that occupational injuries/diseases are inevitable and, therefore, their costs should be borne by the employer as a cost of doing business. In exchange for this, the employee generally is barred from suing the employer under common law. This is usually referred to as the *exclusive remedy doctrine.*

The exclusive remedy doctrine proved to be an equitable solution for both parties. The employer agreed to pay the employee certain benefits (usually medical and income replacement) in the event of an industrial injury or disease. In return for these guaranteed benefits, the employee agreed to give up the right to sue the employer and obtain the large settlements that might result from lawsuits. However, lawsuits may occur in workers' compensation when there is third-party liability, such as a product defect that results in an injury.

Following are the basic objectives of workers' compensation laws:

- To ensure prompt and reasonable benefits to injured employees.
- To relieve public and private charitable institutions from bearing the burden of costs.
- To eliminate, insofar as possible, attorney fees and time-consuming trials.
- To encourage maximum employer interest in safety and rehabilitation through experience rating approaches to premiums.
- To promote research and study in the area of accident causes, with the aim of reducing the occurrence and the human suffering that results.
- To ensure prompt and effective medical treatment to reduce long-term disability.
- To encourage all employers to anticipate and manage on-the-job injuries.

In most states, there are very specific laws governing what types of industrial injuries/diseases are covered. As of this writing, many states exclude job-related stress claims and other mental health disability claims if they are not associated with a physical injury. Multiple chemical exposure claims are also excluded in many states. State laws govern the types of medical benefits to be paid. Alternative medicine and experimental procedures and treatments are often excluded. Some states allow chiropractors to function as attending physicians for injured workers; others do not.

Some states have workers' compensation funds that write coverage for the workers in those states. States with workers' compensation funds may also allow private insurance or self-insurance. The states that have all three types of workers' compensation coverage are called *three-way;* those that primarily or exclusively provide coverage through a state fund are called *monopolistic.*

The benefits under workers' compensation include medical benefits, cash benefits for nonfatal and fatal injuries, and rehabilitation benefits.

Medical Benefits. Medical benefits for covered health care services are payable without limit in most states. Most workers' compensation claims are medical only or involve only the payment of medical benefits. It has been said that because "workers' compensation remains the last stronghold of fee-for-service health care delivery systems in the United States,"[32] case management has great potential for medical cost containment.

Cash Benefits for Nonfatal Injury

Temporary partial disability (TPD)—TPD is an income replacement benefit for a disability that renders a worker temporarily unable to fulfill some of his or her work duties. This type of payment is usually an income supplement for an injured worker who is only able to work part time or in a light duty job that does not pay as well as the job at the time of injury. This type of payment is usually made on a weekly or monthly basis.

Temporary total disability (TTD)—TTD is an income replacement when a disability makes it impossible for the employee to return to work for a given period. This payment is also usually made on a weekly or monthly basis.

Permanent partial disability (PPD)—PPD is for a disability that has a permanent impact on the worker's employability. Workers eligible for this type of award may be unable to work full time or in a job that pays as well as the job at the time of injury. This type of award is generally given as a lump sum at the time the claim is settled.

Permanent total disability (PTD)—PTD is awarded when a worker is unable to return to any form of **gainful employment** for the rest of his or her life. This type of award is usually given in the form of a **pension.**

The majority of states have a waiting period for benefits of, for example, 2 to 3 days before cash benefits are paid. The cash benefits are usually based on a percentage of the wages earned before the disability, with a maximum allowable cap. The purpose of the cash benefits is to replace lost wages while a worker is disabled for an on-the-job injury/disease.

Cash Benefit for Fatal Injuries. Cash benefit for fatal injuries is usually called *survivor benefits* because it is paid to the surviving spouse, children, and/or other family members of the deceased worker. These benefits vary greatly and are subject to various limitations.

Rehabilitation Benefits. Rehabilitation benefits are offered by many workers' compensation systems to assist injured workers in returning to work. These benefits may include vocational rehabilitation counseling, retraining, job placement, assistance with **job modification,** and other services. Rehabilitation benefits may also include case management. The goals of rehabilitation services include (1) appropriate sequencing and coordination of health care, (2) reduction in the amount and expense of litigation, and (3) reduction in the impact of the disability on the worker's ability to return to productive work and, as a result, a reduction in the amount of the permanent partial/total disability award.

Types of Workers' Compensation Programs

State industrial programs—State industrial programs include private insurance, state funds, and self-insured companies. Workers' compensation laws vary greatly from state to state.

Longshoremen and Harborworker's Act of 1972—This federal legislation was enacted to define the workers' compensation benefits for those workers who work on the docks or in the shipbuilding/ship repairing industry (i.e., those who work "on or over the water"). The US Department of Labor's (USDOL) Office of Workers' Compensation Programs (OWCP) regulates those insurance carriers and self-insured employers who administer the program.

Jones Act—The Jones Act governs workers who work on the high seas. Unfortunately, the exclusive remedy doctrine does not apply to this form of workers' compensation, so that the employee must sue the employer in order to gain benefits and coverage.

Federal Employees Compensation Act (FECA)—The FECA was developed to provide coverage to nonmilitary employees of the federal government. It is also administered by the USDOL and the OWCP.

Federal Employees Liability Act (FELA)—FELA was enacted to govern compensation to railroad workers. Like the Jones Act, it does not include the exclusive remedy doctrine, and the worker must sue the employer.

Case Management Services in Workers' Compensation. Case management services are often provided for workers' compensation cases as part of rehabilitation benefits. Usually, the ultimate goal of case management of workers' compensation cases is for the injured worker to return to work in some capacity. Consequently, it is essential for the case manager who has workers' compensation cases to be cognizant of return-to-work issues. These issues are discussed at length in Chapters 20 and 21. They include being able to reconcile the physical requirements of jobs with the physical and mental capacities of injured workers, to assess the work skills and experiences of the injured worker, to assist in modifying jobs or in planning transitional return-to-work programs, and to address safety and prevention issues.

On workers' compensation cases, the case manager will often work closely with the claims adjuster. This will include making recommendations for benefits exceptions for medical treatment, arranging medical **release to return to work,** determining whether the injured worker can return to the job at the time of injury or another job based on transferable skills, and developing a rehabilitation plan if the injured worker must change occupations.

Auto Liability

About half of the states have auto liability; the other half have no-fault. Because of the low dollar limits on policies, auto liability is often not a good source of referrals because the maximum amount is reached quickly in catastrophic cases, and case management is often not warranted as a cost-savings measure. Case management services may be associated with **expert witness** work because of the litigious nature of auto liability and other liability claims. As mentioned previously, case managers may assist attorneys in synthesizing and interpreting medical information. They may also provide case management if hired by the **plaintiff's** (injured party) attorney. Sometimes, they provide life care planning to assist in ascertaining the costs that will be associated with maintaining a severely disabled person for the rest of his or her life and in proper allocation of funding for that purpose.[33]

State funds exist in some states for auto insurance coverage. These often include assigned-risk pools for drivers who cannot obtain regular automobile insurance.

Commercial, General, Product, Malpractice, and Errors and Omissions Insurance

These types of insurance operate much like auto liability insurance does. The most significant difference is that policy limits are likely to be much higher, thus enabling case management to be a more beneficial service. Working in this line of insurance tends to be adversarial because of the litigious nature of this type of coverage.

Auto No-Fault

Individuals who are covered by no-fault insurance receive payment of property damage and bodily injury from their own insurance companies. Sometimes, lawsuits can still be filed if damages exceed certain limits, which usually are established by law. Because auto no-fault laws vary considerably from state to state, whether they are favorable to case management also varies according to jurisdiction.

DISABILITY INSURANCE LINES

Short-Term (STD) and Long-Term Disability (LTD)

LTD and STD are forms of insurance that provide tax-free salary continuance to insured or ill persons who are unable to work because of accident or sickness that is not work related. Medical benefits are not included. STD usually covers disabilities of 6 months or less and may pay higher benefits (sometimes up to 100% of predisability salary) than LTD. Some benefit plans feature a period of STD that is followed by LTD if the claimant is unable to return to work.

LTD usually replaces only about two thirds of income and is capped at a maximum amount. It may also be offset by Social Security benefits, workers' compensation benefits, disability payments provided by travel accident plans, credit disability insurance, pension plans, or retirement plans. LTD benefits tend to vary from carrier to carrier and may extend for the life of the person or to normal retirement age (about 65). LTD coverage may be provided in three different ways:

Group LTD—Group LTD is usually provided through an employer to its employees and generally replaces only two thirds of income and is offset by the benefit plans mentioned previously.

Individual LTD—The terms of the maximum amount of monthly benefit and the maximum period of time for which benefits are payable vary from policy to policy. There are different waiting periods and other terms depending on the applicant's income and occupation. Individual LTD policies pay benefits regardless of any other sources of income, such as for occupational injuries for which the injured person may also receive workers' compensation benefits.

Associated Group LTD—In this situation, an association is the insured, and the members of the association are the ones who are covered by the policy if they pay the designated premium.

Many LTD policies include "his occ/any occ" clauses, which refer to the terms of disability payment under the LTD policy. Generally, for the first 24 months of disability, total disability means the insured (or employee) is unable to perform each and every duty of his or her regular occupation. After the initial 24 months, total disability usually means that the insured is unable to perform any occupation for which he or she has the education, training, or experience.

There is usually a "rehabilitative employment" clause in LTD policies, which allows for the employee to attempt to return to work on a trial basis without jeopardizing the LTD benefits. This clause also allows for the employee to return to work on a part-time basis, with insurance benefits making up the difference between part-time pay and full LTD benefits. There may be funds available for retraining.

Because medical benefits are not paid as part of LTD or STD, case management is used mainly to obtain additional information about the extent to which a claimant is disabled from "his occ/any occ," to assess ability to return to work and to evaluate retraining options. When a case manager is asked to set up an independent medical examiner for this purpose, it may be necessary to perform related vocational services, such as taking the work history, performing a **transferrable skills** analysis, and obtaining **job analyses (JA)** for potential jobs that the claimant may be able to perform by virtue of previous experience or training. The case manager may be expected to perform some of these functions alone or in conjunction with a vocational counselor. (More information about this is included in later chapters.)

SUGGESTED READINGS

Kongstvedt PR: *The managed health care handbook,* Gaithersburg, Md, 1993, Aspen.

Powell SK: *Nursing case management: a practical guide to success in managed care,* Philadelphia, 1996, Lippincott.

Williams SJ, Torrens PR: *Introduction to health services,* New York, 1993, Delmar.

References are found at the end of the book.

CHAPTER 6
LEGAL ISSUES IN CASE MANAGEMENT

Because American society seems to continue moving in the direction of increasing litigiousness, case managers need to be constantly alert for issues and circumstances that might potentially create a situation involving legal liability. Especially, there is potential for legal action in cases where an unfavorable medical outcome is likely to result. Even though case managers do not make medical decisions and their role is of a facilitative nature, the current trend is to name all parties involved on a medical case when a lawsuit is filed, including case managers.[34] Consequently, although physicians make the ultimate decisions on medical care when a case is being managed, the case manager must be sure to take all appropriate steps to ensure that there has been adequate communication among all parties and that informed decisions are being made that take into consideration all variables that are known or should have been known.

This section addresses steps that the case manager can use to ensure that the case is managed appropriately. A number of relevant legal cases that illustrate issues that are bound to arise in the course of case management are cited.

BASIC ISSUES OF GOOD CASE MANAGEMENT PRACTICE

Act first for patient safety—When working with patients, families, and providers, case managers must first consider the safety of the patient in light of the patient's condition and subsequent needs. Whenever there is doubt about what is best for the patient, the case manager must advocate for what appears to protect the patient's safety. If the safety or efficacy of potential therapeutic interventions or placements is in question, the case manager should consult his or her supervisor as well as appropriate medical consultants. Also, if there is a concern that patient safety is being compromised, the case manager may need to take immediate action to secure patient safety, such as moving the patient to another care setting if the current setting represents a potential or real harm.

Function in an advisory role as a case manager—The case manager needs to operate in an advisory capacity in which his or her recommendations are developed to assist the patient, family, and providers in the treatment planning process. None of these parties is bound by the advice given by the case manager, and it is critical that the case manager does not present recommendations as ultimatums or dictates. It is not within commonly accepted practice guidelines for case management to be involved with approval or denial of medical treatment options, as this is the function of utilization review (UR).

Obtain and release medical record information—Case managers must obtain and occasionally release medical record information that is confidential in nature. To operate within federal and state rules and regulations, case management firms need to have confidentiality policies and procedures in place to ensure proper functioning in this area. These policies need to define what kinds of information are confidential and how confidentiality will be protected and secured within the case management firm. These procedures should also include specific instructions on the wording of release forms, the circumstances in which confidential information can be released, and with whom the information may or may not be shared.

Address conflicts of interest—Case management firms, like other entities within the health care delivery system, face conflicts of interest in contract development regarding incentives to overuse and underuse services. For example, if a case management firm enters into a capitated contract for case management services, the financial incentive is to limit the amount of case management services offered to the health plan's subscribers. Conversely, if the case management firm offers its services on an hourly, fee-for-service basis, the financial incentive is to provide as much case management as possible.

In entering into contracts with customers, the case management firm needs to take into consideration how these pricing structures may affect the process of case management. Consequently, case managers need to be willing to fully disclose to patients, families, and providers the nature of their contractual relationships with referral sources so that there is an honest, open working relationship with everyone involved. Case mangers must also be willing to freely disclose who the referral source is and the nature of the relationship between the referral source and the case management firm.

Manage relationships with vendors/providers—In developing contracts or referral relationships or both with providers/vendors, it is important for case management firms to be cognizant of potential price fixing and violations of antitrust laws. Case management firms need to be diligent in assessing the quality of services provided by contracted providers/vendors. They also require some form of ongoing reporting and monitoring of the provider/vendor's performance. There may be some inherent liability involved when case managers channel patients to certain designated providers/vendors. Occasionally, the case manager may be required to use a designated provider network selected by the health plan with no input from the case management firm, but in other situations, the case management firm may be involved in provider/vendor selection. The nature of the relationship with providers and vendors needs to be clarified by the case manager when referrals are made.

Develop collateral materials—When describing the services offered by a case management firm, the collateral marketing materials need to be specific and take into account all of the issues described in this section. General references to "ensuring high-quality care," for example, need to be avoided. The role of the case manager as an independent, advisory facilitator of necessary health care services needs to be emphasized.

Obtain all relevant information—Doing this sounds simple, but there is a dynamic tension between containing costs and ensuring that all relevant information is known. Obtaining information requires expenditures for additional medical tests and evaluations and time for research on the part of the case manager. There is pressure to limit the resources used to obtain information, yet quality of care can be compromised in doing this. This is where the experience, medical expertise, and good judgment of the case manager and any physician advisors who are used as resources come into play. It cannot be emphasized enough that the quality of case management depends on the quality of the case managers and the physician advisors used. Obtaining all relevant information without resorting to unnecessary expenditures involves good judgment based on a thorough knowledge and critical analysis of the pertinent variables on the case.

Use a physician advisor in an appropriate specialty for consultation—When a case manager is faced with a situation that requires additional medical expertise, he or she often will consult a physician advisor in an appropriate specialty. It is the role of the physician advisor to synthesize information for the case manager, so that he or she will have additional knowledge that can be used for such activities as researching other options and communicating or negotiating with the **attending physician** to address issues and consider more cost-efficient alternatives that do not compromise quality of care.

Consult with the treating physician—The treating physician is generally considered to have the most complete knowledge of the patient's situation and is, therefore, usually considered to be the most qualified to make ultimate decisions about a patient's care. Thus, the case manager must always consult with the treating physician and should attempt to thoroughly understand the treating physician's rationale for the treatment plan. At the same time, it is also the role of the case manager to discuss other options with the treating physician. Essentially, the case manager is functioning as a catalyst and resource in the critical analysis and decision making on the part of the attending physician. Ultimately, the treating physician makes the final decision, but the case manager presents options and discusses the case to influence a more informed decision.

Follow procedures scrupulously—Most case management firms have casework procedures that are clearly defined to minimize legal difficulties and ambiguities. These procedures should follow nationally recognized practice guidelines for case management, but they usually are also adapted to take into consideration local issues, such as state laws governing insurance coverage and mandates from referral sources. These procedures should be reviewed and updated, on an ongoing basis to ensure that they address current issues. Procedures should be updated, especially when new case law is written that affects case management and managed care practice. In the rapidly changing world of health care reform, new case law is constantly emerging.

Act timely—Time is always a major factor in medical service delivery and case management. Unnecessary delays cause conditions to worsen, compromise quality of care, and often require increased financial expenditures. As a case manager, you are, in essence, selling your time to the referral source so that medical service delivery to the patient can take place in a more timely, efficient manner. Case managers always need to look for ways of improving and streamlining their involvement to increase the timeliness and efficiency of services.

CASE EXAMPLES

In this section, a number of rules that need to be taken into consideration when working cases are cited. Relevant case law is also cited with some of these rules. Most of these examples are more related to utilization review than to case management, but they are cited here because the underlying principles are relevant to both disciplines.

- *The treating physician's judgment is not conclusive.* A payer has the right to reach its own conclusion on medical necessity using physician advisors and various criteria established from current standards of medical practice. *Sarchett v. Blue Shield of California,* 43 Cal. 3d q, 233 Cal. Rptr. 76 (1987).
- *The treating physician's judgment is nevertheless entitled to great deference.* Because the treating physician has had a longer and more involved relationship with the patient, he or she is generally considered to have a greater knowledge of the facts on the case. *Sarchett.*
- *Utilization review decisions must be consistent with community medical standards. Hughes v. Blue Cross of Northern California,* 215 Cal. App. 3d 832, 263 Cal. Rptr. 850 (1989).
- *Utilization review procedures must be prompt and fair. Wickline v. California,* 192 Cal. App. 3d 1630, 239 Cal. Rptr. 810 (1986); *Wilson v. Blue Cross,* 222 Cal. App. 3d 660, 271 Cal. Rptr. 876 (1990).

WICKLINE CASE

In this case, the patient was covered by the California Medicaid program (MediCal), which included managed care features, such as inpatient precertification and concurrent review. The patient was certified for a specific number of days on a hospitalization for leg problems. Her attending physician believed more days were needed. The Medicaid program cut the number of approved additional days requested in half, and the physician then discharged the patient at the end of that approved time even though the attending physician knew he could request a further extension of Wickline's hospital stay by telephoning the MediCal consultant. Complications developed, and Wickline called her physician to complain of leg pain. Wickline even had an office visit with her physician after discharge, and although there were office notes indicating no substantial change in the patient's condition, the physician could not recall the visit. Ultimately, Wickline was in excruciating pain and was readmitted to the hospital. Attempts to save her leg through the use of various interventions failed. Finally, Wickline's leg was amputated above the knee.

The patient then sued the Medicaid program, along with the providers. The court broadly stated that a third-party payer can be responsible if a defect in the design or implementation of a cost-containment program causes harm. The court went on to say, however, that the treating physician has the ultimate responsibility for his or her patient's care and cannot blame a third-party payer for decisions that are properly the treating physician's.

WILSON CASE

In this case, a Blue Cross member suffered from depression and was admitted to a hospital for treatment. Blue Cross hired an independent utilization management firm, which reviewed the member's hospitalization and said it was not necessary. Blue Cross then refused to pay for further hospitalization, and the member was discharged and committed suicide shortly thereafter. Blue Cross and the utilization management firm were sued and then tried to get themselves dismissed from the case.

The court said the question was whether Blue Cross and the utilization management firm could be said to have caused the member's death.

The court in the *Wilson* case said that the *Wickline* ruling did not let them off the hook in the circumstances presented in *Wilson* and refused to dismiss Blue Cross and the utilization management firm. The court noted that the Blue Cross policy failed to disclose to the member that an independent review firm would be conducting utilization management. The court also relied on the fact that the treating physician wanted the member to stay in the hospital and had stated that he would be alive if he had remained hospitalized. The court said it did not believe that there was any clear public policy favoring private payer utilization management. Based on these factors, the court concluded that Blue Cross and the utilization management firm could be held liable because the decision not to approve or pay for further hospitalization could be viewed as a substantial factor in the member's death.

In contrast to the *Wickline* case, the facts in the *Wilson* case were clear. The treating physician vigorously protested the managed care decision in the *Wilson* case. There was evidence that the parents would have kept the boy in the hospital if they could have afforded it, and the suicide occurred shortly after the refusal to hospitalize, apparently without significant intervening events. The court clarified that the test for causation, where multiple factors lead to the ultimate harm, is whether the **defendant**'s conduct was a substantial factor in causing the harm.

▶ NAZAY CASE

Another case that caused a great deal of concern was *Nazay v. Miller,* 949 F 2d 1323 (3d Cir. 1991). This case involved a self-funded plan with a precertification requirement for hospitalization. Failure to obtain the preauthorization resulted in a reduction of benefits. Mr. Nazay was hospitalized for a heart problem, but he failed to get his precertification, and his benefits were then reduced.

Mr. Nazay sought to have the plan pay the full claim and ultimately brought suit. The district court found that the plan could not include or enforce a precertification requirement in the absence of showing prejudice. This decision was appealed, and the Third Circuit court overturned the district court ruling, holding that an employer could design a self-funded plan as it saw fit and that the plan did not have to show prejudice or harm to enforce the precertification requirement. The court strongly endorsed the right of employers to include and enforce cost-containment measures in their plans.

▶ DUPONT CASE

In the *DuPont v. Sally* case, the court ruled that the payer cannot disregard the attending physician's recommendations for treatment. The payer must show that it has done its own thorough investigation and research into the specifics of the case, such as referral to a utilization management firm. However, the payer, or its designee, cannot totally rely on the treating provider's decision because of the inherent conflict of interest.

▶ HUGHES CASE

In the case of *Hughes v. Blue Cross of California,* decided on March 24, 1988, the California Court of Appeals upheld a trial court's punitive damage awards in compensation against Blue Cross based on a defective utilization management determination of medical necessity.

In this case a California Blue Cross subscriber submitted claims for hospitalizations for her dependent son who had developed mental problems that led to repeated and extended hospitalizations. Blue Cross requested and received the patient's medical records but had only obtained portions of the records. The claim file did not include the hospital discharge summary, records of the patient's treatment at another hospital, or records of the hospital's concurrent utilization review program. The incomplete records were reviewed by a Blue Cross physician advisor who recommended that coverage be denied for two hospitalizations because a lower level of care would have been medically appropriate.

The claim was sent to arbitration, and the arbitrator ordered Blue Cross to pay the claim. Then, the subscriber brought a bad faith action against Blue Cross. The jury awarded compensatory and punitive damages to the subscriber for Blue Cross's breach of its implied covenant of good faith and fair dealing. On appeal, the Court of Appeals upheld the jury's finding that Blue Cross acted in bad faith based on two separate findings:

- First, the court found that Blue Cross employed a standard of medical necessity significantly at variance with community standards to constitute bad faith. It should be noted that the physician advisor reported disapproval decisions in about 30% of the claims he reviewed over several years for Blue Cross.
- Second, the court found that Blue Cross failed to obtain all relevant medical records before the denial of the claim, and this failure to adequately investigate the claim was further grounds to support a finding of bad faith.

SUMMARY

These issues and case examples are presented only as examples and guidelines for case managers, and this is not meant to be used as legal advice. Case management firms need to solicit legal counsel as needed in developing policies, procedures, and contracts.

SUGGESTED READINGS

Carneal G: Any willing provider debate heats up in the courts, *Med Interface* 9(11):109-110, 112, 114, 1996.

Gnessin AM, Carroll SV: Recent regulations clarify the application of Medicare fraud and abuse legislation to managed care relationships, *Med Interface* 9(5): 110-112, 114, 1996.

Hogue EE: LegalEase, understanding laws, rules, regulations: tips make CMSA standards work for you, *Case Management Advisor* 6(6):75-76, 1995.

Hogue EE: Are case managers liable? *J Care Management* 1(2):35-38, 53, 1995.

Reference is found at the end of the book.

PART II

Practical Aspects of Case Management

CHAPTER 7

CASE IDENTIFICATION, REFERRAL, SCREENING, AND AUTHORIZATION

The appropriate identification of cases for case management is a concern to many referral sources because if cases are not properly screened, cost containment will not occur. Some screening methods identify too many cases for case management. When cases with limited potential to benefit from case management are referred, cost savings are not realized, and costs on the claim may even increase because of the fees that accrue from case management services. Conversely, if case management screening criteria are too stringent, cases with potential to benefit will not be identified for referral, and cost containment will not occur. (See Appendix 1 for examples of case management screening criteria.)

The development of appropriate screening criteria for case management should be a major focus of any company that wishes to provide case management services. Some referral sources have their own screening criteria to handle this function internally, but many referral sources expect this service from the case management companies they use. (See Appendix 1 for examples of criteria.)

Many health insurance claims with potential to benefit from case management are identified through UR as part of precertification and continued stay review. Occasionally, cases are identified through a retrospective review program. When a claim is screened for an admission or continued stay, usually sufficient information is also obtained to assess its potential to benefit from case management. Companies that provide these UR services generally have custom software programs that also screen automatically for case management. If the precertification or continued stay review screening identifies the case for case management, the UR nurse will coordinate the case for additional screening.

For other lines of insurance (such as workers' compensation), UR may not be used proactively. Workers' compensation carriers or self-insured employers often expect the case management provider to provide free screening of cases, which is usually done as part of a file review that may take place at the referral source's office. This may also take place at the case manager's office if a copy of the file is faxed or mailed. This type of screening is often performed on a subjective basis by the case manager using her or his experience and medical expertise. More and more, however, case management companies are using objective, written criteria to screen cases.

SCREENING CRITERIA

What criteria to use for case management screening is a big issue for many companies providing case management regardless of whether they use a computerized system for screening or perform this function manually. Some of the criteria apply equally to all cases, but some criteria are developed in response to local issues, such as state legislation governing workers' compensation, Medicaid, and so on, and specific needs of individual referral sources. One main type of criterion is diagnosis. Many screening systems contain a list of severe or catastrophic diagnoses that usually benefit from case management. These diagnoses often include the following:

- Head injuries
- Spinal cord injuries
- AIDS or HIV-related conditions
- Severe burns
- High-risk neonates
- Organ transplants
- Psychiatric conditions
- Oncology

Other criteria include the following:

- Age of patient
- Multiple admissions or claims for same condition
- Multiple diagnoses
- Psychologic factors
- Multiple providers
- Adequacy of facility or treatment
- Lifestyle considerations
- General health status
- Social factors

(See Appendix 1 for examples of case management screening criteria and a case management referral screening criteria form.)

OBTAINING APPROVAL FROM REFERRAL SOURCE

Regardless of the method of screening, once a case has been identified for case management, approval may have to be obtained from the referral source if the case manager is to proceed with case management. Before contacting the referral source for approval, it is standard practice for the case manager (or other person who obtains referrals for the case management company) to write up a referral form (see Appendix 2 for example of form). The referral form should contain all the pertinent information about the case that is required to open the file for case management and begin working the case. This information includes demographic information as well as the reasons and goals for the referral.

It is important for the case manager to pay special attention to the reasons for referral section on the referral form. This should clearly indicate the expectations that both the case manager and the referral source have regarding how the case is to be worked. In some respects, this serves as an informal contract between the referral source and the case management company about what services are authorized and what goals are to be achieved.

The referral form is generally presented to the referral source or is mailed or faxed, and a copy is kept by the case management firm for the case file. Because time is of the essence in managing many cases, **authorization** to proceed with case management usually is obtained over the phone or in person during file reviews that take place at the office of the referral source. Authorization should be obtained as quickly as possible on catastrophic injury cases because many of the decisions that affect expenditures and quality of care are made during the first few days following the incident. It is important to document the authorization for the referral, including hours and activities authorized, for clarity and to expedite payment for case management services.

At the time a referral is made, the case manager should also request copies of any medical reports or records that are in the referral source's files. Sometimes, especially on health insurance cases, the referral source will have no records. At other times, notably workers' compensation cases, the files may contain extensive records. It is always valuable to perform a review of any records that are available before beginning work on a case.

QUESTIONS TO ASK THE REFERRAL SOURCE

When working with different referral sources, it is important to remember that each line of insurance has different goals and expectations for case management. Questions that it may be helpful to ask to clarify issues that may arise during the course of working the case include the following:

- Are benefits exceptions made if cost savings can be demonstrated?
- Who (at the referral source) is responsible for making authorizations? Are there different levels of authorization?
- If the case is workers' compensation, are the issues on the case primarily medical or vocational?
- Is contact with the employer necessary or appropriate? Under what circumstances?
- How long will benefits last? Are there any dollar limits on benefits?
- What types of exclusions and limitations are listed in the benefits package?
- Are there any special eligibility issues (e.g., COBRA)?

SUGGESTED READING

Strassner LF: The ABCs of case management: a review of the basics, *Nursing Case Management* 1(1):22-30, 1996.

CHAPTER 8
ON-SITE VERSUS TELEPHONIC CASE MANAGEMENT

ON-SITE CASE MANAGEMENT

Case management services may be performed telephonically or on-site. It is estimated that telephonic case management went from 15% of all cases in 1990 to 85% in 1995.[35] **On-site case management** involves personal visits to the client/family, attending physician, employer (on workers' compensation cases), and others who may fulfill crucial functions in the management of the case. This is the traditional method of conducting case management, and it tends to be more effective than telephonic case management, although it is usually much more costly.

Advantages of On-Site Case Management

With in-person visits, it is often possible to explore issues in more depth than one can do in a phone call. In-person visits with health-care providers allow for the quick exchange of written reports and other materials (such as x-rays) that have to be in hand to be used. Personal visits can be more effective for assessment, education, exploration of issues, problem solving, and negotiation.

Sometimes, crucial elements of the case cannot be identified except through a personal visit. For example, a client always appears clean and well groomed when his physician sees him at the office. When the case manager visits the client at his home, she observes that it is filthy and contains many potential sources of infection with which the client could come into contact while he still has open wounds from a surgical procedure. This issue can be discussed with the client during the home visit, and an action plan can be developed to address the sanitation problems in a satisfactory manner.

At times, multidisciplinary team meetings and staffings on the client are valuable for the case manager to attend. Often, case managers meet with clients in physicians' offices to discuss problems and reach solutions that are mutually agreeable to all parties. Multidisciplinary treatment programs often have staffings that the case manager must attend because he or she is also a member of the treatment team who must fulfill certain functions for the client to derive maximum benefit from the program. In-person meetings with the client and family are often the most efficient ways of performing the educational role that case managers are so often required to fulfill. Educational meetings not only allow for the involvement of multiple persons, but they also permit the use of charts, diagrams, videos, and other audiovisual aids.

On-site visits are more intimate in the sense that they convey to the client/family that someone is taking a personal interest in his or her medical progress. This can be extremely important to a family in crisis because one of its members has had a catastrophic injury or sudden medical emergency. In-person visits also create the impression that the referral source is interested in the well-being of the client as well as saving medical dollars. Quality of care issues can often be addressed more effectively on-site, where the case manager has the opportunity to observe what is actually going on. Likewise, it is sometimes easier to resolve certain problems when all parties involved can observe the situation and, therefore, have accurate information about what is truly happening. This is especially true with psychiatric or behavioral issues that are often ill-defined and have vague causation.

On-site case management also involves a lot of telephonic work to be cost effective. When contemplating an on-site visit, the case manager always needs to examine whether a visit will produce results that are not likely to be obtained through other methods of case management (i.e., telephone calls or correspondence). Even though on-site case management is authorized on a case, in-person visits always need to be made judiciously and sparingly. Occasionally, only one visit is made to the client/family, and the rest of the case is worked telephonically.

Another factor that differentiates the two types of case management is report writing. On-site case management usually requires narrative progress reports that are written monthly. Telephonic case management may not include comprehensive narrative reports, although various outcome data on telephonic cases may be reported statistically, often in aggregate reports.

Disadvantages

Although on-site case management has all of these factors to recommend it, the main drawback it has is cost. In-person visits are usually quite costly because of the travel time and expenses involved. Occasionally, phone calls can substitute quite effectively for on-site work. Many times, the benefits of in-person work have to be balanced against the cost effectiveness of telephonic case management.

Because case management is often used as a cost-containment measure, case management companies have to be cognizant of the costs they incur through provision of their own services. This is especially true if the potential for saving dollars through case management is low. On the average, except in working with referral sources whose main area of focus is quality of care, the cost savings achieved through case management need to be lower than the costs of providing case management services. For this reason, some cases are best handled telephonically.

TELEPHONIC CASE MANAGEMENT

In **telephonic case management,** all services are provided over the phone or through correspondence, faxes, e-mail, or electronic transfer. This saves considerable time, thereby reducing the overall cost of case management. It also allows the case manager to handle a larger caseload and the referral source to provide case management services to more clients, thus improving the quality of care for more individuals and controlling costs on more cases.

These factors allow for more efficient use of resources that may be scarce (i.e., qualified case managers and funding to provide medical benefits to subscribers or recipients).

Some of the services provided telephonically include interviewing the client/family, employer, and physician to assess needs and develop a plan for implementing case management, coordination of services, comparison shopping for service providers and medical equipment, discharge planning, researching and negotiating benefits exclusions, and negotiating prices with providers. Sometimes, when cases are managed telephonically, there is no direct contact with the subscriber/client/recipient. In general, on-site case management tends to be more thorough, more global and addresses more client issues. Telephonic case management may be limited to one small aspect of the case, such as discharge planning or locating an appropriate treatment facility in the client's geographic location.

Comparison of Telephonic with On-Site Case Management

Telephonic case management tends to proceed in a more rapid fashion than the on-site variety. Because of this, telephonic case management often tends to be used when quick decisions have to be made on a case. Discharge planning is a case in point. The case manager does not usually have time to visit the client/family and the attending physician to discuss the case because the client needs to be discharged as soon as possible. Unnecessary days of inpatient care are extremely costly.

On the other hand, on-site case management is very valuable when the recovery period is anticipated to be somewhat lengthy, quick decisions do not have to be made, and time must be allotted for evaluation, consideration of options, negotiation, and trial and error. Workers' compensation cases often fit into this category because the client is usually not being cared for in an inpatient setting. Different job options at the employer at time of injury need to be considered. The client may need to participate in a transitional return to work plan and may have to undergo a work hardening program to develop the physical stamina to return to work safely.

On-site case management is also useful for catastrophic injuries because the recovery period is lengthy, necessitating many medical decisions along the way. Because multiple medical providers are often involved on catastrophic cases, it is often helpful to have multidisciplinary staff meetings (that may include the client and family) so that all players are aware of the issues on the case and what each person is doing to bring about improvement or recovery.

Some referral sources determine that all of their cases are to be case managed either onsite or telephonically. Some use a mixture of on-site and telephonic case management, which they may determine themselves, according to the type of case or treatment modality, or leave to the discretion of the case management provider. When the type of case management to be used is to be determined by the case management firm, a careful analysis of the cost benefits to the case of both types of service modalities needs to be made.

Some referral sources have preconceived ideas about whether case management should include in-person visits. Consequently, whenever a referral is received from a new source that has not specified whether it prefers in-person or telephonic case management, the case manager should always clarify whether site visits are authorized. Likewise, if it becomes clear

BOX 8-1

CRITERIA FOR ON-SITE VERSUS TELEPHONIC CASE MANAGEMENT

The following criteria are helpful in deciding which cases are more suitable for on-site versus telephonic case management.

ON-SITE CASE MANAGEMENT

Case is catastrophic
Dollar limits are high
Many treatment providers and other interested parties are involved
The patient/family requires education and individual counseling
Observation of the patient is desirable
Attending physician or other treatment providers are unresponsive

TELEPHONIC CASE MANAGEMENT

Referral source is concerned about cost containment
Case is likely to be short term and noncatastrophic
No case manager is located in patient's area
Case manager has already established good rapport with treatment providers
Rapid decision making needs to take place
Dollar limits and time frames are short
Patient/family have good communication skills

Appendix 1 at the end of this book provides additional information on telephonic versus on-site case management screening criteria.

that a site visit is warranted on a case that is being managed telephonically, the case manager should always obtain authorization before proceeding. With some referral sources, on-site visits may never be authorized regardless of how valid the reasons for them may be.

SUMMARY

When establishing a case management program, firms need to decide whether they will provide telephonic or on-site case management and what criteria they will use for recommending each service (see Box 8-1; also, see Appendix 1 for examples of telephonic and on-site case management screening criteria). Because of the scarcity of resources and increased recognition of the value of case management services, telephonic case management seems to be on the increase. This allows for the use of this service on a larger number of cases, although it may be less effective overall in some respects.

Case managers need to be trained on effective techniques for telephone use to accomplish difficult tasks that might be better accomplished in person. Assertiveness training and negotiation skills are two areas that are beneficial to case managers. Similarly, case managers need to be trained on how to get the most from in-person visits and how to judge when they are warranted.

SUGGESTED READING

Romaine DS: Case management challenges, present and future, *Continuing Care* 14(1):24-31, 1995.

Reference is found at the end of the book.

CHAPTER 9

INITIAL ASSESSMENT, INTERVIEWING, AND COUNSELING SKILLS

INITIAL ASSESSMENT

Once a case management referral has been received and any records accompanying it have been reviewed, the case manager will perform an **initial assessment** to develop a plan of action for case management activities. As discussed in Chapter 10, this assessment may be extensive and may include in-person visits to the client/family, attending physician, employer (on workers' compensation cases), and others, or it may be accomplished through telephone calls to pertinent individuals. Regardless of the method used, good counseling and interviewing skills are required.

Most case management firms have basic forms the case manager may complete while interviewing the client/family, attending physician, other medical providers, and employer. These forms contain most of the relevant information that needs to be obtained to work the case. Separate forms may be used to interview the client/family, medical providers, and employer. Most companies adapt the forms they use to suit the needs of their referral sources. Some even have separate forms for different referral sources or lines of insurance, most notably, workers' compensation and health insurance. (See Appendix 2 for examples of initial interview forms for client/family and health care provider.)

If the case is being managed on-site, the case manager may address all of the issues on the forms during in-person visits. Since telephonic case management may be limited to one discrete element of the case, such as discharge planning, the case manager may complete only pertinent parts of the interview form, or a special interview form may be developed for discharge planning only.

It is important to complete the pertinent sections of these forms while conducting the initial assessment interviews. These forms help to organize pertinent information and assist the case manager in being thorough in considering all factors that have a bearing on the case.

Deciding What Information to Obtain

The general information obtained in an initial assessment with the client/family includes the medical history of the client, the client/family's perception of the prognosis, treatment, and progress, and nonmedical factors that may affect the case. Whether or not to include the family in the initial assessment is a judgment call for the case manager. Sometimes, the family needs to be very actively involved in the treatment of the client and plays an active role in decision making. At other times, the case progresses better if the case manager works with the client alone. Some families are highly supportive and fulfill crucial roles in the care, treatment, and recovery of the client. If the client is unable to make decisions about medical care and treatment, the case manager must work with the family. There are families, however, who exert an undue negative influence on the client. They may pressure the client into making decisions that are not in his or her best interest, or they may assume an overprotective role that impedes progress by taking away independence. The case manager must use his or her judgment regarding how to most effectively work with the family to achieve the best results for the client.

The information to be obtained from medical providers includes diagnosis, history of the current illness or condition, review of systems, psychosocial status, prognosis, projected discharge date, discharge needs, patient compliance, and other factors. When there are multiple providers, the case manager has to decide whether to interview all of them. This is also a judgment call. Providers who are no longer treating the client will probably not need to be interviewed unless they have some crucial information that cannot be obtained elsewhere. The providers who are most essential to include are those who will be making decisions and recommendations on the case, such as discharge date, discharge needs, treatment regimens, necessary medications, further surgery, referrals to other providers, and release to return to work.

Interviews with employers that take place on workers' compensation cases often focus more on vocational issues than medical ones, although the line between the two often is blurred. The main issue to be explored with an employer is if the client can safely return to work in any capacity. This involves a determination not only of whether the client has the physical capacities to perform jobs that are available but also of whether the client possesses the vocational skills required. This subject is discussed at length in Chapters 20 and 21 on vocational evaluation and rehabilitation.

Evaluating the Information Obtained

Once the interviews (in-person or telephonic) have taken place, the case manager needs to evaluate the information that has been obtained. If there are gaps in information, the case manager needs to develop strategies to obtain what is missing. This may consist of recontacting some of the major players in the case, or it may involve setting up appointments for IMEs or other medical assessments. The case manager must also determine what goals need to be achieved on the case and how they can be achieved. For example, the goal may be for a client with cancer to be discharged from the hospital to a **hospice.** To implement this goal, the case manager may have to research hospices that are located in the city where the client lives. If the insurance policy does not cover hospice care, the case manager may have to research the costs of in-patient care for the client as long as he or she is projected to live versus hospice care. The case manager may then use these facts to discuss a benefits exception with the carrier.

Developing appropriate recommendations after the initial assessment can be particularly challenging for new case managers. It is easier and safer to spend a great deal of time writing summary information, but it is more difficult to clearly state what the case manager will do as a result of all the medical, insurance or benefit plan, psychosocial, vocational, financial, and other relevant information that has been gathered. A supervisor may need to assist the case manager in developing appropriate recommendations, and the referral source may want to be contacted by phone to discuss possible recommendations before receiving the written report. The case manager must keep in mind that the referral source may need to pay for benefits exceptions and other costs associated with the recommendations contained in the initial assessment report.

Case management recommendations should include the goals and objectives from the case management activities. The responsibilities and actions that have to come from others, such as the client or the referral source, should be described in the recommendations section, especially if the report is shared with these individuals. All the people, facilities, and agencies who are affected by case management need to understand what the goals are, what actions are being taken, and what their respective roles are in the process. This helps to ensure successful case management outcomes because everyone knows what is expected in this type of collaborative approach.

With on-site case management, the case manager may write a narrative initial assessment that reports and discusses all the pertinent issues on the case and makes recommendations for future case management services. For telephonic case management, the case manager may contact the carrier by phone to discuss what needs to take place and obtain approval to proceed with it. Sometimes, this may involve some form of brief written report that is faxed or transmitted electronically because time usually is a factor in telephonic case management. Since the goal of saving inpatient days requires very timely work, the case manager would use whatever methods are at his or her disposal to obtain approval for hospice care as soon as possible. Even though a formal, written report would not be made, the case manager might fax some written information about the hospice and its costs versus inpatient care to the carrier.

How to write a narrative, initial assessment report is covered in Chapter 11 on report writing.

INTERVIEWING SKILLS

Interviewing is a fine art that goes far beyond merely obtaining responses to a series of questions. Often, the person interviewing does not know what some of the most pertinent issues are. If he or she sticks to a predetermined list of questions, some of the most significant factors on the case may not come to light. The art of interviewing is in getting the client/family or other individuals to talk freely about their concerns. Although these skills can be used in interviewing anyone, they will be focused primarily on working with the client/family. Professionals who are being interviewed usually do not require or have time for as much rapport building or discussion of the role of the case manager.

Before any interview can begin, the case manager needs to establish rapport with the person being interviewed. The client/family may not have any familiarity with the role of the case manager and may be apprehensive that the case manager is concerned only with the interests of the insurance company. Consequently, one of the first steps in establishing rapport is to explain the role of the case manager. This explanation should emphasize that the case manager is an objective third party who is bound by a code of ethics to ensure that the client receives safe, necessary medical treatment in an appropriate setting. The client/family should have the opportunity to ask questions and express concerns about the function of case management. The case manager should be prepared to answer questions about her or his professional background, areas of expertise, and reimbursement method from the referral source.

Special emphasis must be placed on empowering clients/families to make their own decisions. The case manager needs to acknowledge that the ultimate decision will be made by the client/family, probably in consultation with the attending physician, but that the case manager's role is to facilitate informed decisions by providing accurate information and addressing issues that are of concern. Some other techniques for rapport building include making small talk, expressing concern about the client/family's situation, and paying compliments. However, these techniques should not detract in any way from the professional purpose of the interview and the professional image of the case manager.

Although the case manager has a baseline of information that needs to be obtained, direct questions are not always the best way to obtain it. Direct questions are appropriate for factual information, such as, "What medications are you taking?" or "How long did your doctor say your recovery period would be?" However, direct questions often do not produce much information on such things as feelings, worries, conflicts, dilemmas, and other issues that are somewhat nebulous and that people are often reluctant to discuss directly.

These issues can often be inferred from the content of other comments that the person being interviewed makes. Successful interviewing requires good listening skills to pick up issues that the client/family may be reluctant to discuss directly. When these issues are expressed indirectly, the case manager may facilitate further discussion on them by reflecting back to the client what was expressed and letting the client know that further elaboration would be acceptable. For example, a client may say, "I have been getting lots of medicine from Dr. J., that old pill-pusher." The case manager might facilitate further discussion by saying, "That old pill pusher?" This comment on the part of the case manager reflects back to the client what he or she said and requests more clarification by phrasing the client's comment in the form of a question. In this way, the case manager can address such issues as whether the client is having symptoms of being overmedicated or feels that the attending physician should be considering other options besides medication.

When asking questions that do not require a factual answer, it is helpful to phrase them in such as manner that they will obtain an open-ended answer. Some examples of factual questions are: "How old are you? How much do you weigh?" Examples of open-ended questions are: "What do you think needs to take place for you to get well? What other medical conditions might you have that could be interfering with your recovery?"

Although this discussion is focused primarily on working with the client/family, there are some techniques that are valuable in interviewing medical providers and employers. Since these individuals usually have much more decision-making power than the case manager, it is wise at the beginning to acknowledge their role as the major decision maker. When facilitating decisions on the part of the medical provider or employer, the case manager must be armed with an accurate and thorough arsenal of information on the options that are available. The most persuasive tool with professionals usually is comprehensive information that overwhelmingly supports the option that is the best choice for everyone concerned. However, the information presented must be objective and needs to take into consideration that the medical provider may have additional information that is not available to the case manager. All interviews, negotiations, and information sharing with medical professionals must be objective and oriented toward what is best for the client, not the referral source.

COUNSELING SKILLS

One of the most important counseling skills has already been mentioned—active listening. One cannot provide counseling without understanding the client's issues and concerns. This requires the ability to listen to the objective content of what the client says, the implied content, and the emotional tone that accompanies the content.

In discussing what other counseling skills besides listening are required, it is helpful to explore what counseling is not. First and foremost, counseling is not advice giving. Advice is generally only given when the client asks for it or when the counselor has an ethical obligation to warn the client that some untoward event will result from an action that is taken or not taken. Counseling may involve the exploration of options, but the counselor does not advise the client on which option to take. Counseling also is not problem solving or a mere discussion of an issue or problem. It is a much more active process, although it may involve problem solving at times.

One of the reasons why counseling is not primarily problem solving or advice giving is that its focus is client empowerment. The purpose of counseling is to aid the client in making better decisions, taking control of his or her life, understanding his or her feelings and motivation better, and acquiring the knowledge and skills to overcome difficulties. The emphasis is on helping the client learn to appraise situations, seek out information, identify options, and make informed choices based on these options. Giving advice circumvents this client empowerment model and leaves the decision making and power in the hands of the counselor or other professionals with whom the client is working.

There are many theories and methods of counseling that have been developed in this century. Basically, most methods will fit into one of two categories—directive and nondirective. Some methods incorporate both categories. Most case managers will find it useful to use both methods at different times with different clients while working on cases but will most often use directive techniques.

Nondirective Couseling

In nondirective counseling, the counselor adopts a role that appears passive to the client. The counselor allows the client to discuss whatever he or she wishes and does not attempt to guide the subject of the conversation. Although the counselor appears passive, he or she is actually engaging in active listening. The role of the counselor in nondirective counseling is to listen to what the client says and to reflect it back in ways that help the client to clarify what has been expressed. The purpose is to help the client to contemplate what has been expressed and to come to some resolution about it.

A brief example illustrates how nondirective counseling works:

Client: *Sometimes I feel so angry that I had this stupid accident. Why do I have to pay for someone's silly mistake for the rest of my life? I am suffering and no one seems to notice or care about how I feel.*

Counselor/case manager: *It sounds like you have a lot of anger about the accident and feel that no one really understands your suffering.*

Client: *Yes, my doctor doesn't care at all. He won't even write me a prescription for pain killers. He just tells me to take aspirin and Motrin. He must think it is all in my head. He only gives me two minutes of his time and tells me to go home and shut up.*

Counselor/case manager: *You seem to feel that your doctor is not doing all that he can to help you. You also seem to feel that over-the-counter pain medication is not helping.*

Client: *I need something stronger to relieve the pain, but my doctor won't give it to me because he thinks I will become addicted.*

Counselor/case manager: *You feel your doctor is not responsive to your request for pain relief, and you are not sure about what to do about this situation.*

Client: *Maybe I should see another doctor and discuss having surgery.*

Counselor/case manager: *You are considering surgery as a possible option to help reduce your pain.*

Obviously, nondirective therapy can be an extremely time-consuming process for a case manager who is trying to empower the client to make some positive choices regarding his or her treatment options. It also has the disadvantage of relying heavily on the client's knowledge of options that are available in making choices. In the example above, the case manager is relying on the client to come up with possible courses of action, but the only ones the client seems to be aware of are pain medication and surgery. Obviously, the client needs more information than is usually supplied by the counselor using a nondirective approach.

However, using a nondirective approach has some advantages in the example above. The client is exploring his feelings in a nonthreatening manner, and the case manager is obtaining some valuable information about the client's relationship with his attending physician that she might not otherwise see if a more directive approach was used.

Directive Counseling

Directive counseling is a more active method in which the counselor imparts information, presents options, and gives opinions on what is discussed. A directive counseling session might proceed like this:

Client: *My doctor doesn't seem to care whether I get well or not. He doesn't really do anything except ask me how I am feeling when I go to see him.*

Counselor/case manager: *Thus far, your doctor has been treating you conservatively with bed rest, icing, anti-inflammatories, and muscle relaxants. Have you discussed physical therapy or surgery with him?*

Client: *I brought up the subject of surgery once, but he said I wasn't a good candidate for it because I smoke and because of my age. He thinks that I should try conservative treatment first. He sent me to a physical therapist, but I only went once because the exercises hurt so much that I had to spend the next day in bed.*

Counselor/case manager: *Did you tell the physical therapist how much the exercises hurt? Have you considered going back to physical therapy, discussing the pain caused by the first session, and seeing if the therapist can modify the exercises so that you won't hurt so much but the same effects can be achieved?*

In this session, the case manager is not giving advice or making decisions for the client but is actively exploring options to empower the client to make some choices that may assist him in his recovery. The case manager is much more active in asking for information from the client and presenting options for the client to consider. In the nondirective scenario, the case manager does not ask for information specifically and guides the client in identifying options rather than presenting them directly.

Clearly, a directive approach to counseling is more likely to achieve the goals of case management in a timely manner. As a health care expert, the case manager's role is to educate the client. This is difficult or impossible using a nondirective approach. However, the case manager may wish to be nondirective when dealing with feelings or hidden agendas that the client may not wish to discuss openly.

Directive counseling often takes a behavioral approach. This means that the focus is on assisting the client to change behaviors that are maladaptive or need improvement in order for the client to be well adjusted and healthy and to be able to participate fully in life. One of the premises on which this type of counseling is based is that the client's feelings, beliefs, and attitudes will change if there is a corresponding change in behavior. More positive behaviors will generate reinforcers internally and from the environment (such as feeling better, having more energy, making new friends) that will help the client to change his or her feelings and beliefs. New behaviors often help the client to have improved self-esteem as well.

A behavioral approach is often helpful in case management, particularly when client/family education is being provided or when the case involves psychiatric or substance abuse treatment. A behavioral approach generally involves educating the client on the advantages and disadvantages of changing certain behaviors. Often, the case manager will find it helpful to develop a behavioral contract with the client. With a behavioral contract, the client and case manager reach a mutual agreement about behaviors and courses of action that are to be carried out by both the client and the case manager. These contracts can be either verbal or written and signed by both parties. The case manager must use his or her own judgment regarding which type of behavioral contract to use. Generally, verbal contracts are used first because written contracts tend to make the relationship between the client and the case manager adversarial.

Behavioral contracts in case management are often used when the client is not complying with the treatment program (e.g., not taking medication, missing medical appointments, not doing a home exercise program) or is engaging in behaviors that are detrimental to recovery (e.g., doing heavy lifting, not staying in bed).

BOX 9-1

EXAMPLE OF A WRITTEN BEHAVIORAL CONTRACT

CLIENT

I, [client's name], agree to the following:
I will take one tablet of [medication name] three times a day.
I will do the home exercise program prescribed by [physical therapist's name] every day.
If I am unable to keep an appointment with the case manager, [doctor's name], or [physical therapist's name], I will call to reschedule with 24 hours advance notice, if possible.
I will attend the **work hardening** program every day for 2 weeks.

CASE MANAGER

I, [case manager's name], will do the following:
I will arrange for a panel examination for [client's name].
I will meet with [employer's name] to discuss a transitional return to work program that will involve part-time work to start and a reduction in lifting requirements.
I will research the adaptive equipment that is available to reduce the amount of weight lifted and overhead reaching on the job and will negotiate with the insurance carrier to purchase any that seems appropriate.

As workers' compensation cases tend to be adversarial because the client must cooperate or lose income replacement benefits, written behavioral contracts may be used more often. These contracts may include both medical and vocational issues. To make them less adversarial and one sided, they often include sections on the obligations of the case manager and others involved with the case. Box 9-1 presents an example of a written behavioral contract.

In this example, the expectations of both the client and the case manager are clearly spelled out so that there will be no misunderstandings of what each is supposed to do in order to achieve the goals of the case management plan. In line with the goal of client empowerment, which must always be kept in mind in counseling, behavioral contracts are always developed in conjunction with the client. They are never written just by the case manager and presented to the client to sign.

Clients who are not motivated to participate are always difficult to handle in a counseling situation. For some individuals, there are many incentives for remaining disabled, such as income replacement for not working, being absolved of responsibilities, increased attention from family members, and enjoyment of the sick role. Often, the case manager must work with the client/family in counseling to identify the incentives for remaining disabled and must develop a behavioral contract with the client/family to overcome these barriers. A positive approach is usually recommended, but, unfortunately, sometimes the best incentives to get clients to cooperate and participate are negative consequences (such as a reduction in benefits) for noncompliance.

A comprehensive discussion of counseling techniques is beyond the scope of this book. Case managers who have not had training in counseling as part of their education should acquire additional training.

SUGGESTED READINGS

Brown SD, Lent RW: *Handbook of counseling psychology,* Somerset, NJ, 1992, Wiley.

Loughary JW, Ripley TM: *Helping others help themselves: a guide to counseling skills,* Blacklick, Ohio, 1979, McGraw-Hill.

Lovett H: *Cognitive counseling and persons with special needs: adapting behavioral approaches to the social context,* New York, 1985, Praeger Paperback.

CHAPTER 10
WORKING THE CASE

Cases are worked in a variety of ways depending on whether they are telephonic or on-site, but both types of cases have as their foundation a case management plan. Indeed, the first step following the initial evaluation is to write the case management plan. Some referral sources may want a formal, written plan that has to be approved before it is carried out. For many cases, this will not be necessary, but it is still important for the case manager to have a basic, written plan to guide him or her by defining the goals that need to be achieved and organizing the steps that need to be taken to reach them.

DEVELOPING A PLAN

The first step in plan development is defining the goals that are to be achieved. Some goals may be very simple, such as moving the client from the hospital to the home. Other goals may be more complex. Often, on catastrophic cases, there may be a long-range goal (such as independent living and return to work) and a number of short-term or intermediate goals (e.g., speech therapy, relearning **activities of daily living (ADLs)**, obtaining a prosthesis, obtaining appropriate transportation) that have to be reached to make progress toward the long-term goal. In developing goals, it is usually beneficial to start with the ultimate or long-range goal and break that into intermediate or short-term goals. Because case management is traditionally oriented toward saving medical dollars, some of the goals may be financial (e.g., negotiating a reasonable rate with a treatment facility that meets the client's needs, teaching the family to provide care to the client so that home health care is no longer needed, comparison shopping and negotiation to obtain the best prices on durable medical equipment).

Establishing Goals

To establish goals for the client, the case manager must consult with the client's attending physician and, sometimes, with other health care providers. Occasionally, a client may be in a treatment facility that has a multidisciplinary team that meets regularly to discuss client progress and establish and reevaluate goals. The case manager may need to be part of these multidisciplinary teams. The case manager will influence decisions made by the team, and the team will help to establish goals that the case manager will execute. If the case is workers' compensation, the employer at the time of injury may also be involved in establishing goals, such as the type of work to which the client may return or whether the client will be provided with modified work on a transitional or permanent basis. The client's family may also be involved in goal setting, particularly if they will have to provide care for the client on either a temporary or a permanent basis. If the client is not competent to handle his or her own affairs, a **guardian ad litem** may be a major player in any goals that are established.

The referral source will also have its own goals that will need to be addressed in conjunction with the goals of the other parties on the case. The goals of the referral source will most likely be to close the claim, to save dollars on the claim, and, on workers' compensation cases, for the client to return to work. Some referral sources, such as Medicaid, also have maintenance of quality of care as a major goal.

Most importantly, the client and the family need to be empowered to take an active role in goal setting. Progress toward any goal is most likely to be made if the client has made an informed choice to participate in the goal. All goal setting must be made in conjunction with the client/family or his or her representative. Often, it is beneficial to have three-way conferences with the client, attending physician, and case manager. These conferences allow all participants to express their concerns and issues so that decisions can be reached that are agreeable to all parties. Similarly, clients often participate in interdisciplinary team meetings. The goal is to assist the client in becoming aware of all the issues on the case and to help him or her to make informed decisions. Having client buy-in is critical to the success of any medical treatment plan or any other program that is developed as a part of case management. Unless the client is empowered to act on his or her own behalf in making informed choices and feels that his or her needs have been addressed, the client will function essentially in a passive role in which the medical providers or the case manager is expected to bring about recovery. Generally, the best results are obtained when the client assumes a major part of the responsibility for recovery.

Over and above improving the chances for recovery, the client must always be treated with respect and dignity. This involves recognizing that the client is a free agent and, ultimately, is the one who will be most affected by any decisions that are made. Consequently, one of the most important goals of case management is empowerment of the client to make informed choices that are based on accurate information and careful weighing of the advantages and disadvantages of pursuing various courses of action.

Conflicting Goals. At times, the goals of the various health care providers, the client, the family, and other involved persons will conflict. One of the major roles of the case manager is to function as a mediator among the various individuals on the case so that a consensus can be reached on goals.

Because of conflicting goals, it may take some time and a number of contacts with the different parties on the case to establish what the long-range and short-range goals will be. Often, goals can be established with only telephonic contact; at times, formal meetings are required.

Determining How Goals Should Be Achieved. An important component in establishing goals is determining how they are to be achieved. Obviously, if a goal is not achievable, it should not be chosen. Thus, the goal development process also involves developing a plan for achieving the goal. Sometimes, tentative goals are set, but on further research, it is discovered that they are unrealistic or cannot be achieved in quite the way that had been anticipated. When this happens, it is necessary to revise goals in view of new information on the case. On long-term cases, goals frequently are revised on an ongoing basis as new information surfaces. Even on short-term cases, the case manager must be flexible enough to change courses frequently if necessary. Flexibility is a most important characteristic to have in working any case because things often do not go as anticipated.

Good problem-solving skills and creativity are also paramount. "Case management problems require creative problem solvers who use *productive thinking.* Productive thinking generates a new solution for each new problem. In contrast, *reproductive thinking* reuses an old solution to solve a new problem. . . . Experienced case managers use both productive and reproductive thinking, breaking with old problem-solving habits and solutions when new problem situations occur."[36]

Thus, the written case management plan must contain both long-term and short-term goals and a list of services or other entities that are required to achieve them. What is needed to achieve goals will usually include treatment modalities or procedures, medications, possibly new care providers or facilities, services that the case manager will perform, and medical evaluations. On workers' compensation and LTD cases, vocational rehabilitation services may also be included (e.g., retraining, job modification, job placement).

Pricing Considerations. In identifying what is needed to achieve goals, prices must also be included. Many of the items that are identified may have to be authorized by the referral source. This is especially true if benefits exceptions are to be made. As the case manager works the case, he or she needs to always be cognizant of the fact that one of the ultimate goals of case management is to achieve dollar savings on medical costs while maintaining quality of care. Because of this, the case manager always needs to be price conscious and aware of whether any goals or recommendations are likely to save money and how much. At the conclusion of the case, the case manager will be expected to assess the outcome of case management, including how much money was saved through case management.

Pricing negotiations with health care providers need to be coordinated with the claims payer, so accurate claims submission can result in prompt payment.

The process of establishing goals and the means to achieve them is an ongoing process throughout the case. The case manager must remain in close contact with the referral source, client/family, attending physician, and other appropriate health care providers at all times in order to keep the case moving and to obtain authorizations for services as necessary. The attending physician and the referral source are the main players in obtaining authorizations that are sought on an ongoing basis.

The Role of Research in Goal Development. Goal development and action plans for achieving them often require extensive research. This research is made through conferring with medical providers on the case, co-workers, and physician advisors, accessing the Internet, consulting various reference books and other sources of written information, and contacting facilities, agencies, and other community resources. This subject is explored more fully in Chapter 12 on researching medical issues during casework.

Much of the work on any case takes place by telephone to save time. Visits are made as needed but are usually infrequent because one of the goals is to save money, which includes controlling the costs of the case manager's services.

PREPARING THE REPORT

Report writing is a significant part of working cases from many referral sources. For a variety of reasons, it is important to have information clearly documented in writing. Consequently, progress reports are generally written on a monthly or bimonthly basis. These reports describe what has happened on the case since the previous report and make recommendations for future services that may have to be authorized by the referral source. More information on report writing is contained in Chapter 11.

Timely reports can be a major factor in referral source satisfaction with case management. Reports allow the referral source to assess whether case management is effective, and they present information that is essential for making decisions, such as benefits exceptions. Reports also document the services that have been provided by the case manager and document his or her billing. Essentially, the report is the only tangible product that the case manager has because the referral source is unable to directly observe the services that have been provided and the results obtained. Therefore, it cannot be emphasized enough that good reports are an essential element of case management services delivery. Timely, well-written, informative reports are one of the best marketing tools there is because they depict what has taken place on the case and the results obtained.

As well as writing reports, the case manager needs to have phone contact with the referral source at appropriate intervals. Sometimes, other written correspondence is needed besides reports. This will vary by referral source. Because some referral sources like to be contacted frequently and others prefer minimal contact, case managers must learn their preference. When making contact with a referral source, it is important to remember that every phone call, letter, or report is a marketing opportunity. Referral sources are impressed by the professionalism of case managers. They are not impressed by case managers who complain or do not seem to know what they are doing. A frequently voiced concern is that case managers call referral sources to ask what to do on a case. Referral sources refer cases for case management because they do not have the expertise to manage them inhouse, and they do not want to be asked what to do because they believe that is what they should be getting from case management.

This does not mean, however, that case managers should not ask for authorization to proceed with certain services or that the opinion of the referral source should not be sought when choices are to be made among various options. Referral sources generally appreciate it when case managers give them a choice of options to be pursued and describe the advantages and disadvantages of each option.

CLOSING A CASE

There comes a time in every case when goals have been adequately reached or other factors indicate that sufficient progress has been made that case closure is appropriate. Case managers need to be alert to this so that they can recommend case closure to the referral source. It is important to involve the referral source in the decision to close the case because the referral source may have additional courses of action that it wishes the case manager to pursue.

Sometimes, the decision to close the case is based on the perception that the case has progressed as far as it can go and that further case management services will not be benefi-

BOX 10-1

CRITERIA FOR CASE CLOSURE

The decision is made jointly between the client and the case manager based on the following:

- Further services not warranted or cost effective
- Patient nearing **maximum medical improvement**
- Goals met and no further goals identified
- Policy or benefit limits have been reached
- Patient has reached stop-loss under initial customer's plan and case referred to reinsurance
- Patient loses eligibility for coverage
- Customer requests closure

cial. It is important to be able to recognize when this occurs because case management has been criticized as being an add-on service rather than a cost-containment service (see Box 10-1). If services continue to be provided when they are no longer cost effective, case management may actually increase costs rather than reducing them.

Often, a closing report is written that details what took place on the case and what results were achieved by providing case management. This subject is addressed more fully in Chapter 19 on outcomes management. The closing report is an important marketing tool because it informs the referral source of the benefits of case management on that particular case and cases in general.

Much more can be said about working the case, and many of these issues are covered in their own, separate chapters. Most of the services and other components that go into case management occur simultaneously and cannot be separated into discrete factors. Case management is a complex job that involves being able to attend to many different issues and considerations at the same time. The case manager must be able to play many roles and must be flexible enough to adapt to working in many unfamiliar situations with individuals who have many different viewpoints and agendas.

SUGGESTED READINGS

Coleman JR: New challenges call for rewriting the rules for problem solving, *Case Manager* 7(2):47-50, 1996.

Mullahy CM: Case managers and physicians: working associates not adversaries, *Case Manager* 3(2):62-66, 1992.

Mullahy CM: *The case manager's handbook,* Gaithersburg, Md, 1995, Aspen.

Powell SK: *Nursing case management: a practical guide to success in managed care,* Philadelphia, 1996, Lippincott.

Retzlaff K: Dollars and sense: what to know when choosing your medical equipment provider, *Continuing Care* 10(9):20-21, 25-26, 1991.

St. Coeur M, ed: *Case management: practice guidelines,* St. Louis, 1996, Mosby.

Tips from the field, uncovered services: ask corporate executives to pay, *Case Management Advisor* 6(4):53-54, 1995.

Reference is found at the end of the book.

CHAPTER 11
WRITING CASE MANAGEMENT REPORTS

Case management reports may follow a variety of formats. Each case management firm probably will develop its own report writing formats to address the needs of the services it provides and the needs of its customers. Some customers, especially government agencies, will have their own report writing formats that must be followed if one is a contractor. Other customers, such as insurance carriers, may also have very specific formats that they have developed to provide them with the written information they require. Sometimes, the signatures of clients and their attending physicians must be obtained for a case management or rehabilitation plan in order to show agreement and commitment to the goals and recommendations.

This manual contains basic report writing formats in Appendix 2 at the end of the book that can serve as a guide for locally developed formats. They contain all the elements usually required in case management reports. These templates can be used as-is or modified to meet the needs of individual cases and specific referral source requirements. Separate templates are provided for medical/surgical cases and psychiatric/**chemical dependency services.** This chapter addresses both the essential elements that should be in most reports and general report writing considerations that will assist the case manager in producing well-written, professional, informative reports.

GENERAL CONSIDERATIONS

The most important thing to remember about report writing is the medical expertise level of the referral source. Normally, claims adjusters may have limited medical backgrounds. If the person who will be reading your report does not have a medical background, it is important to use layperson's terms and thoroughly explain all terminology that someone with limited medical expertise would not reasonably be expected to understand. The general rule on this is that it is better to overexplain than underexplain. The case managers who write the best reports remember that "the nature of the referral source or payer will subtly affect communications from the initial assessment through the reporting stage."[37]

However, as insurance personnel normally have heavy workloads, it is important to write reports that are short and to the point and contain no unnecessary information. Some case managers, in an effort to be thorough and meticulous, write reports that are many pages long. Unfortunately, their attention to detail is often for nought because their reports do not get read. When faced with a lengthy document and limited time, many individuals only read the summary and recommendations. Therefore, case managers should pay most attention to the summary and recommendations sections. In general, all information that is essential for the referral source to know should be incorporated into the summary and recommendations.

Writing style should be somewhat terse but should be readable and professional. Clients should be referred to as "Mr." or "Ms." Only children should be referred to by their first names. Even though excess verbiage should be avoided, complete sentences always should be used. To avoid the appearance of bias, events or characteristics should always be described in behavioral terms. It is all right to offer your opinion about what is going on in the case, but this should only be done following a description of an event or situation that illustrates your opinion. In general, reports should contain more than just factual information. They should contain action plans based on events taking place on the cases.

In writing reports, as in all writing, it is better to "show" rather than "tell." Reports need to be very specific about who, what, when, where, and how.

A brief example will illustrate these points:

Improperly written report: *Susan does not want to be seen for a psychiatric evaluation by Dr. E. because she has had bad experiences with him in the past. Therefore, I have made an appointment for her to be seen by another psychiatrist.*

Better report: *Ms. A. has missed three appointments for a psychiatric evaluation with Dr. E. Each time she postponed her appointment, she stated that she was ill or did not have anyone to babysit for her four children. According to a report from Hospital Z where Ms. A. was treated briefly as an inpatient, "she does not like Dr. E. and does not feel that he listens to her or takes her needs into consideration." After Ms. A. postponed her third appointment, the case manager became concerned that she would not meet with Dr. E. in a timely manner and would not derive maximum benefit from the evaluation because of her stated feelings toward Dr. E. Therefore, the case manager decided to make an appointment for Ms. A. to see Dr. H. instead. This is scheduled for January 3 at 9:00 AM.*

In this example, the improperly written report refers to the client by her first name and merely gives an opinion about the client's motivation without describing any behaviors that would lead to that conclusion. The improperly written report also does not indicate who the new psychiatrist is and when the appointment will take place (who and when).

In the better report, the case manager describes some behavior on the part of the client that led to the conclusion that seeing Dr. E. was probably not the best course of action in the opinion of the case manager. As a result of the events described and the conclusions that could be drawn from them, the case manager decided to change the plan and have the client see a different psychiatrist.

Whether to refer to oneself in the first or third person in reports is always a subject of controversy. Reports written entirely in the third person (i.e. "in the opinion of the case manager . . .") sound more professional and academic, but they are somewhat dry to read. Using the first person is more friendly and informal and makes the report more readable. Generally, it is not wise to shift back and forth between the first person and the third because it tends to confuse the reader.

Another area of controversy is whether to use the passive voice or action verbs. The passive voice is generally used in professional and academic writing, but it is also dry. Action verbs give any writing more punch and readability. Perhaps the best reports use a combination of passive voice and action verbs to convey professionalism but not at the expense of readability.

Reports should always be written in a tactful manner when describing conflicts, differences of opinion, or misconduct on the part of any of the parties involved on the case. Disrespectful statements and value judgments are to be avoided even if one or more of the parties involved was clearly in the wrong.

When writing reports and recording information in patient files, it is important to remember that clients may be able to legally access and read what has been written. Sometimes, laws will buffer this by requiring that a professional be in attendance to answer questions and provide explanations when the client is reading his or her own file. Occasionally, patients are permanently barred from reading files containing psychiatric and other types of information, but it is best to assume that patients will be able to read any information included in their files. If it is necessary to put something in a report that should not be read by the patient, the report should contain a prominent notice to that effect.

A case manager should always stay within his or her areas of expertise when writing reports. Case managers should not make diagnoses. For example, a report might state that a client "has smelled of alcohol every time he has been seen by the case manager." This would be a proper behavioral observation, but if the report went on to say that the client "is an alcoholic," the case manager would be making a diagnosis that was beyond his or her scope of expertise.

One reason for writing a report is to justify the extent and billing of case management services. In other words, the report should contain a summary of the case that indicates what activities the case manager performed and are being billed to the referral source, but this need to justify billing has to be balanced with brevity. As mentioned previously, reports should not contain excess detail that makes them too lengthy. One way to avoid excess detail yet describe what services were delivered is to enclose case notes or a contact sheet with the report. A contact sheet or case notes (see Appendix 2 for example) will list the activities performed on the case during the reporting period, the date they were performed, and the time and expenses associated with them.

Reports are generally written to cover billing periods (e.g., once a month). Each report should summarize the activities that took place during the billing period just completed and should make recommendations for activities that will take place during the next billing period. Recommendations should be written in specific, behavioral terms that state who, what, when, where, and how, and they should be numbered sequentially according to the order in which they will take place. They should also indicate how much time will be needed to complete all recommendations and list a diary date for the next report. The following are examples of poorly written recommendations and well-written ones:

Poorly written recommendations: *Make appointment for a psychiatric evaluation. Send paperwork to psychiatrist to complete.*

Well-written recommendations:

1. *The case manager will contact Dr. H.'s office to obtain an appointment for a psychiatric evaluation for Ms. A. within the next 2 weeks.*

2. The case manager will send job analyses for accounting clerk and claims clerk I to Dr. H. for approval and signature by the end of the month.

Estimated time for completion of all recommendations: 2.5 hours.

Next report date: January 27, 1997.

The poorly written recommendations are vague in a number of respects. They do not indicate who will be carrying them out, specifically what will be accomplished, and who will be involved (e.g., name of psychiatrist).

Information that was contained in previous reports should not be repeated in subsequent ones. Referral sources often complain about reports repeating what they already know and about having to pay for duplication of services. In the same vein, case management reports should also not repeat what is contained in reports from other professionals except for a brief summary that describes the rationale for the action that the case manager took based on those reports.

The book *Elements of Style* by William Strunk and E.B. White[38] may be helpful if you experience difficulties with grammar, sentence structure, and punctuation.

MEDICAL/SURGICAL CASE REPORTS

Initial Assessment

The initial assessment should include critical elements, some of which are described in the paragraphs that follow.

Reason for Referral. All initial assessment reports should begin with a summary of the reason(s) for referral. This lays the groundwork for the case and the initial assessment by describing what is to be achieved through case management.

Diagnoses. Next, the primary and secondary diagnoses should be listed and described, with particular attention to their severity.

Facilities. List all facilities in which the client has been confined within the last year, with the addresses, telephone numbers, and dates. Be sure to describe the types of facilities.

Health Care Providers. List all physicians, psychologists, chiropractors, and other providers, with their addresses, telephone numbers, and specialities. Be sure to indicate the primary or attending physician.

Brief History of Current Illness. Describe in a short paragraph the history of the current illness, including complications, reason for admission, and current treatment plan.

Current Medical Status. Describe and assess the current medical status of each, or at least the involved major organ system, paying special attention to the ones involved in the condition(s) that are being case managed. You will also need to describe potential and actual complications that result from the disease or illness. You may need to research the condition(s) in reference materials, or you may need to consult with a physician advisor who has expertise in the area. If there are no current problems or potential complications, that should be indicated. The organ systems that may be addressed include the following:

- Neurologic/psychiatric system
- Gastrointestinal system
- Visual and auditory systems
- Cardiovascular system
- Pulmonary system
- Integumentary system
- Genitourinary system
- Musculoskeletal system
- Endocrine system

Note: Although these systems may be addressed, the case manager may want to use less technical language when doing so to show sensitivity to the level of medical expertise of the reader.

Psychosocial Status. Describe here the family or marital situation, including any dependent children or adults. Discuss the client's marital status or primary relationship and how that affects the recovery process. Describe also the client/family's view of the condition and how realistic they are regarding the recovery process. This section should also contain information about compliance with treatment and your assessment of the client/family's ability to cope with the medical condition and how strong the support system is.

Care and Equipment Cost Analysis. Discuss the current care and equipment that are being used and whether they are medically necessary. The hospital billing office can give you room charges and equipment charges. You need to itemize the equipment and state whether it is rented or purchased and make recommendations for more cost-effective acquisition of equipment if appropriate. This section should also discuss care alternatives, with prices that would reduce costs as well as improve the quality of care for the patient. It may be helpful to list or make a chart of alternatives and their prices to assist the referral source in making cost comparisons.

Savings. Based on your previous analysis, you need to recommend how savings can be realized. If you are unable to document savings at this time, tell the referral source what you need before you can make such recommendations, such as a meeting with the attending physician. You will also need to discuss how savings can be realized through preventive measures, such as patient education. This section should address current savings, short-term savings (less than 1 year), and long-term savings (over 1 year).

Goals. Describe the treatment goals and strategies that you, the attending physician, the client/family, and others have developed.

Summary and Recommendations. All pertinent aspects of the case need to be summarized here along with recommendations for specific case management activities.

Contact Sheet. This includes a listing of all case management activities and expenses for the reporting period.

Monthly Case Management Update

This report is written on a monthly basis to update the referral source on activities or progress that has taken place on the case since the last report. This report contains essentially the same elements as the initial assessment report except that the referral summary, diagnosis, facilities, health care providers, and history of current illness sections may not have to be repeated. Current medical status and psychosocial status are combined and summarized in a current medical/psychosocial status section. The monthly update or progress reports should contain new information and should not repeat information from previous reports.

PSYCHIATRIC AND CHEMICAL DEPENDENCY CASES

These reports are written in much the same way as medical/surgical reports, with the exception that under current status, the case manager will use the multiaxial evaluation system developed by the American Psychiatric Association as described in the *Diagnostic and Statistical Manual of Mental Disorders—IV (DSM-IV)*.[39] The first three axes and, if possible, all five should always be addressed by the attending physician. Also indicate the principal diagnosis and include a brief explanation of this system if the referral source is unfamiliar with it.

According to the *DSM-IV*, the "multiaxial system involves an assessment on several axes, each of which refers to a different domain of information that may help the clinician plan treatment and predict outcome."[40] In describing the severity of a disorder, the case manager may use such terms as "mild," "moderate," "severe," "in partial remission," "residual state," and "in full remission." These terms are defined as follows:

Mild—Few, if any, symptoms in excess of those required to make the diagnosis; symptoms result in only minor impairment in occupational functioning or in usual social activities or relationships with others.

Moderate—Symptoms or functional impairment between "mild" and "severe."

Severe—Several symptoms in excess of those required to make the diagnosis; symptoms markedly interfere with occupational functioning or with usual social activities or relationships with others.

In partial remission or residual state—The full criteria for the disorder were previously met, but currently only some of the symptoms or signs of the illness are present. "In partial remission" should be used when there is the expectation that the person will completely recover (or have a complete remission) within the next few years, as, for example, in the case of Major Depressive Episode. "Residual state" should be used when there is little expectation of a complete remission or recovery within the next few years, as, for example, in the case of Autistic Disorder or Attention-Deficit Hyperactivity Disorder. ("Residual state" should not be used with Schizophrenia, since by tradition there is a specific residual type of Schizophrenia.) In some cases, the distinction between "in partial remission" and "residual state" will be difficult to make.

In full remission—There are no longer any symptoms or signs of the disorder. The differentiation of "in full remission" from "recovered" (no current mental disorder) requires consideration of the length of time since the last period of disturbance, the total duration of the disturbance, and the need for continued evaluation or prophylactic treatment.

The following are descriptions of the five axes and how the case manager should describe the client's current status and complicating factors.

Axis I (Clinical Disorders, Other Conditions That May Be a Focus of Clinical Attention)—Axis I is used for "all the various disorders or conditions in the Classification except Personality Disorders and Mental Retardation (which are reported on Axis II.)[41] There may be multiple diagnoses needed to describe the current condition on Axis I (e.g., Psychoactive Substance Use Disorder and Mood Disorder). The diagnosis as exhibited by the client should be discussed, as should the treatments, medications, and therapies being used. Long-term complications should also be included.

Axis II (Personality Disorders and Mental Retardation)—This axis is used for disorders that generally begin in childhood or adolescence and continue without change into adult life. These features are not true of Axis I disorders.

In some instances, there may be no disorder on Axis I, but the reason for seeking treatment is limited to the condition noted on Axis II. If this is the case, Axis II should be indicated as the primary diagnosis. If there is no Personality Disorder, Axis II can be used to describe personality traits or common defense mechanisms. The case manager should describe how the Personality Disorder or Mental Retardation will affect the treatment plan, as well as the effect of the long-term outcome of the case.

Axis III (General Medical Conditions)—This is the section where the case manager may list and describe any medical conditions and how they affect the recovery process. If there is no Axis III diagnosis, this needs to be indicated.

Axis IV (Psychosocial and Environmental Problems)—Use of this axis is optional. The types of psychosocial and environmental problems should be listed, such as death of spouse, loss of job, change of school. Psychosocial and environmental problems may include the following:

- Problems with primary support group
- Problems related to the social environment
- Educational problems
- Occupational problems
- Housing problems
- Economic problems
- Problems with access to health care services
- Problems related to interaction with the legal system/crime
- Other psychosocial and environmental problems.[42]

In general, the case manager should describe how this category will have an impact on the treatment plan and long-term recovery.

Axis V (Global Assessment of Functioning)—This axis allows for overall evaluation of the client's psychologic, social, and occupational functioning based on the Global Assessment of Functioning Scale (GAF Scale). The GAF Scale score can be grouped in the following way[43]:

100-91	Superior functioning in a wide range of activities.
90-81	Absent or minimal symptoms.
80-71	If symptoms are present, they are transient and expectable reactions to psychosocial stressors.
70-61	Some mild symptoms or some difficulty in social, occupational, or school functioning.
60-51	Moderate symptoms or moderate difficulty in social, occupational, or school functioning.
50-41	Serious symptoms or any serious impairment in social, occupational, or school functioning.
40-31	Some impairment in reality testing or communication or major impairment in several areas, such as work or school, family relations, judgment, thinking or mood.
30-21	Behavior is considerably influenced by delusions or hallucinations or serious impairment in communication or judgment or inability to function in almost all areas.
20-11	Some danger of hurting self or others or occasionally fails to maintain minimal personal hygiene.
10-1	Persistent danger of severely hurting self or others or persistent inability to maintain minimal personal hygiene or serious suicidal act with clear expectation of death.
0	Inadequate information.

If the current GAF score is available, the case manager may wish to discuss how it compares with GAF scores of the past year as an indicator of the client's ability to recover.

Before working with these classifications, the case manager should become familiar with the *DSM-IV.* This manual should be part of the reference library of any case manager who intends to work with psychiatric and chemical dependency cases.

The Current Medical Status section is eliminated in reports on psychiatric and chemical dependency cases. The Psychosocial Status section is replaced with a Family and Other Psychosocial Factors section, which contains basically the same information except that the issue of abuse and neglect in the home environment is also a subject of focus. The Care and Equipment Cost Analysis section is replaced with a Care Cost Analysis section that addresses costs of care in the current treatment setting and care alternatives that would reduce costs as well as ensure quality of care for the client. Costs of current treatment should be compared with the costs of alternative types of care available.

COMPUTER-GENERATED OR AGGREGATE REPORTS

These reports are usually developed so that the referral source can obtain statistical data on the effectiveness of the case management program. To generate these types of reports, a case management firm needs to have a data or information management system to record and sort pertinent data required by referral sources. Some examples of these types of reports are cost savings reports, aggregate reports by diagnosis, and case manager and functional outcomes reports.

CONFIDENTIALITY ISSUES IN REFERENCE TO REPORTS

The right to privacy is a cherished tenet of democracy in the United States. With modern technology, people are becoming increasingly concerned about who has access to their records and how certain knowledge may be used against them or may cause them public humiliation and missed opportunities. Because most documents created in the course of managing cases can be subpoenaed and, thereby, may become a matter of public record, case managers need to pay attention to what they include in reports. Of particular concern is information or opinions that cannot be substantiated or that the case manager does not have the professional expertise to make.

SUGGESTED READINGS

American Psychiatric Association: *Diagnostic and statistical manual of mental disorders—IV,* Washington, DC, 1994, Author.

The Chicago manual of style, ed 14, Chicago, 1993, The University of Chicago Press.

Mullahy CM: *The case manager's handbook,* Gaithersburg, Md, 1995, Aspen, pp 161-169.

Strunk W, White EB: *Elements of style,* New York, 1979, Macmillan.

References are found at the end of the book.

CHAPTER 12

CREATIVITY IN RESEARCHING MEDICAL AND OTHER ISSUES DURING CASEWORK

It cannot be emphasized enough that case managers need to be able to research medical issues but they do not need to be experts on every medical condition they encounter. This is especially significant on cases with multiple injuries or disease processes occurring simultaneously. Often, beginning case managers who consider themselves experts on certain conditions (e.g., high-risk neonates or orthopedic injuries) feel inadequate if they have to take a case that is out of their area of expertise or if the client has another significant condition that they do not know much about. At other times, the case manager takes the case but is not sure how to efficiently obtain needed medical information. The case manager may be afraid that he or she will miss essential issues of concern on the case because of not knowing the appropriate questions to ask. Not managing the case properly because of inadequate or missing information can be a case manager's worst nightmare.

Other issues besides medical ones may also need to be researched. These include pertinent legislation and rules and regulations of the referral source, nonmedical community resources, and nonmedical concerns that may affect the recovery process (e.g., domestic violence, cultural and ethnic issues, options for retraining).

SOURCES OF INFORMATION

When a case manager encounters a medical or other situation that he or she does not know much about, there are several ways of obtaining needed information in a manner that is cost efficient for the referral source. The method chosen will depend on what is needed, the resources available through the case management firm, and how much time can be billed to the referral source for research-related activities. The most frequently used research methods are described in the discussions that follow.

Consulting with a Supervisor or Other Case Managers in the Firm

Often the best sources of information that are the quickest to access are co-workers within one's own firm. There may be other case managers who have had special training or experience with the issue of concern. Sometimes, generalist case managers are also good sources of information because they have worked many different types of cases and know where to go to find written resources. Co-workers or a supervisor may be able to answer specific questions or direct you to written information in an expeditious manner. These individuals may be consulted whenever the need arises, and information can be obtained in a much more timely and efficient manner than using reference books or on-line sources.

Consulting with Physician Advisors

Many case management companies, especially those that also provide UR, have **physician advisors** on staff or working in a consulting capacity. These physicians are usually **board certified** or **board eligible** and also have their own practices so that they remain current in the field. Like co-workers, physicians can provide a relatively fast and efficient means for obtaining information and advice on cases. Every case management company should consider having physician advisors on a contract basis for consultation on difficult or complex cases. These physician advisors should be in specialties that are related to the most frequent types of cases that are seen by the case management company. For example, if the case management company does mostly workers' compensation work, the physician advisors should be orthopedic surgeons, physiatrists, or neurologists, as workers' compensation cases involve mostly orthopedic and soft tissue injuries.

Reference Books and Other Written Materials

Every case management company should have a library of basic reference books that can be used by case managers as they go about their daily business. These need to be kept in a central location so that they are available for use by everyone who needs to use them. These books may include some of the common references used by medical personnel and are listed in Box 12-1.

As well as having medical reference books, case management companies also need to have other references that relate to the type of services provided and the referral sources served. These may include the following:

- Policies and procedures manuals and codes of regulations from referral sources.
- Copies of state and federal regulations.
- Vocational rehabilitation reference books (e.g., *Dictionary of Occupational Titles, Occupational Outlook Handbook, Guide for Occupational Exploration, Selected Charac-*

BOX 12-1

COMMON REFERENCES USED BY CASE MANAGERS

Physician's desk reference (PDR), most recent edition, Montvale, NJ, Medical Economics.
Blakiston's pocket medical dictionary, ed 3, New York, 1973, McGraw-Hill.
The Merck manual of diagnosis and therapy, most recent edition.
Fischback F: *A manual of laboratory and diagnostic tests,* ed 4, Philadelphia, 1992, Lippincott.
Kirschner CG and others: *Physician's current procedural terminology (CPT),* ed 4, Chicago, 1992, American Medical Association.
Melonakos K: *Saunders pocket reference for nurses,* Philadelphia, 1990, Saunders.
Sherman JL, Fields SK: *Guide to patient evaluation,* ed 3, Garden City, NY, 1978, Medical Examination Publishing.
St. Anthony's ICD-9-CM: code book for physician payment, Alexandria, Va, 1993, St. Anthony Publishing.
Taber CW: *Taber's cyclopedic medical dictionary,* ed 8, New York, 1961, McGraw-Hill.

teristics of Occupations, Classification of Jobs, The Revised Handbook for Analyzing Jobs).

- Journals and periodicals. *The Case Manager, Continuing Care, Journal of Care Management,* and *The Case Management Advisor* are all excellent journals to subscribe to. There are also a number of insurance periodicals, such as *Business Insurance,* that contain valuable information. Certain types of medical and nursing journals may also be helpful. More and more periodicals of this type are being published.
- Books and references on insurance and government agencies, such as Medicare and Medicaid, that serve as health care purchasers.

Following are other written materials to have on hand or keep on file.

- Most recent brochures from health care facilities or agencies and other treatment providers (e.g., head injury programs, skilled nursing facilities, home health agencies, panel examiners).
- Brochures from nonmedical, social service providers (e.g., shelters for the homeless, Meals-on-Wheels, credit counseling services, parenting programs, educational programs, job training facilities, employers).
- Files of job analyses, lists of employers, and labor market surveys (see Chapter 20 on vocational rehabilitation for further information).
- Files of completed health care facility/agency questionnaires. (These can act as a starting point for further research into appropriate facilities and agencies. Be sure to verify all information if some time has elapsed since the questionnaire was completed.)
- Files on medical providers for setting up independent medical examinations and making referrals for such services as physical therapy. (These files are usually based on the experience of the case managers at the firm.)
- Files of special instructions from referral sources.

On-Line Databases and CD ROM

Much information can be accessed from on-line databases, such as MEDLINE. With the advent of the **Internet,** considerable information of all sorts is available to those who know how to move about in cyberspace. More and more medical databases can now be purchased on CD ROM. The modern case management company would do well to keep current on what is available from these sources and provide appropriate computer equipment with convenient and easy access to them.

Public Libraries, College and University Libraries, Medical Libraries, and Law Libraries

All of these types of libraries are excellent sources of information, although it may be somewhat time consuming to visit them to do research.

CASE MANAGEMENT SERVICES THAT REQUIRE EXTENSIVE RESEARCH

Legal consulting, expert witness work, and life care planning all require extensive research. In legal consulting, attorneys may ask a case manager to do research in addition to reviewing, synthesizing, and making recommendations on medical reports on personal injury cases. The research may have to do with such issues as whether two seemingly unrelated medical conditions have a common etiology or if a specific medical procedure or treatment is considered experimental or unproven regarding its effectiveness.

Expert witness work may require research to determine what would be accepted nursing practice in a given situation. Research of this nature may involve surveying nurses and agencies that provide nursing services to ascertain what their policies and procedures or criteria would be.

Life care planning requires research into what kinds of treatments, services, supplies, equipment, and other assistance (e.g., vocational training, transportation, housing) are needed to maintain the client for the rest of his or her life when a catastrophic injury or condition exists. This may involve research into the course usually associated with the medical condition as the person ages, including complications and associated conditions that are likely to develop. Once the course of the medical condition is known, the case manager needs to research what kinds of treatments, services, supplies, equipment, and other assistance may be needed and their costs in today's dollars. Because a number of books and training programs have been devoted to life care planning, no more than rudimentary information is given on it in this book.

Case managers who wish to do life care planning and other expert witness work would do well to accumulate as many professional certifications and other qualifications as possible. This includes the CCM, CRC, or CDMS designations, bachelors or masters degrees, authorship of professional publications, and clinical experience. In doing expert witness work, "the first step to convincing a jury to award your client the funds to implement a care plan is to convince jurors that you are a qualified expert witness."[44] The more credentials you have, the more difficult it is to impeach the fact that you are qualified to testify as an expert.

Another aspect on which to focus is making a good impression in court based on your appearance and the professionalism of your demeanor. "You can be the No. 1 expert on rehabilitation in the country, but if you don't look believable your client may not get his funding."[45]

SUGGESTED READINGS

Deutsch P, Weed R, Kitchen J, Sluis A: *Life care plans for the head injured: a step by step guide,* Orlando, Fla, 1989, Paul M. Deutsch Press.

Deutsch P, Weed R, Kitchen J, Sluis A: *Life care plans for the spinal cord injured: a step by step guide,* Orlando, Fla, 1989, Paul M. Deutsch Press.

Taking your case (management) to court, *Case Management Advisor* 6(5):73-74, 1995.

Team approach energizes life care plans, *Case Management Advisor* 6(3):33-34, 39, 1995.

Weed R, Field T: *The rehabilitation consultant's handbook,* revised ed, Athens, Ga, 1994, Elliott & Fitzpatrick Vocational Services.

Weed R, Sluis A: *Life care plans for the amputee: a step-by-step guide,* Orlando, Fla, 1990, Paul M. Deutsch Press.

References are found at the end of the book.

PART III
SETTING UP A CASE MANAGEMENT PROGRAM

CHAPTER 13

MARKETING CASE MANAGEMENT

One of the first steps in setting up a case management program is to research the marketplace to obtain information on potential markets for case management. This information forms the foundation for any case management program because it determines what kinds of services will be provided to targeted referral sources. With this information, a case management firm can develop programs that will address the needs of the system(s) in which it plans to work. Knowledge of the marketplace will determine the qualifications of the case managers to be hired and will serve as a framework for actual service delivery.

Once the marketplace has been researched, appropriate business plans have been crafted, and appropriate program(s) have been developed, active sales and marketing activities are initiated to secure business, but it is not necessarily the most significant factor in retaining it. Likewise, marketing is not always the most essential element in company growth. Over the long run, service excellence tends to be more significant than marketing in sustaining company growth. Because of this, every case manager needs to approach casework as constant and ongoing marketing. Indeed, service excellence is always the best form of marketing.

LEARNING WHAT POTENTIAL REFERRAL SOURCES EXPECT

Companies that are just developing a case management program need to meet with potential referral sources to learn what their issues, concerns, and expectations are. In the early days of case management, referral sources did not know much about case management, and they tended to trust the expertise of the firm from whom they purchased services. In recent years, however, the industry has matured considerably, and referral sources have become much more sophisticated in their knowledge and expectations of case management services. Now, referral sources have their own ideas about how case management can benefit them. Instead of selling referral sources on the idea of generic case management, firms must now ask referral sources what their needs are and what goals they hope to achieve by incorporating a case management program. Being able to listen and to act accordingly are key issues.[46]

Competition among case management firms is increasing all the time. Referral sources have a wide array of services from which to choose. Sometimes, they find it difficult to identify which case management firms will best meet their needs because none is an exact fit. The firms that most closely address the needs of referral sources tend to be the most successful.

Marketing now requires more listening to referral sources to learn about their expectations from a case management program. For a new program just starting out, this may involve interviewing potential referral sources before even establishing concrete ideas for a case management program. Referral sources often have very specific expectations about such things as qualifications of case managers, billing, reporting, and how the case is to be managed. Learning about these expectations in the beginning may save the case management firm from making costly errors and potentially alienating referral sources by not giving them what they want.

Because of the diversity of referral sources, firms that are beginning to market case management need to be well versed in insurance, managed care, cost containment, and other terminology to be able to confer with referral sources in a meaningful manner. It is also important to be knowledgeable about applicable state and federal laws, especially when attempting to access workers' compensation systems, the Veterans Administration, CHAMPUS, and Medicaid. A primary marketing strategy needs to be "let's figure out together where your problem cases are so that we can work together to manage them to meet your corporate goals."[47] The emphasis has to be on working together to address the needs of the referral source rather than merely attempting to sell them on what the case management firm has to offer.

Communicating in this way with potential referral sources will assist the case management firm in identifying potential markets for their services and in tailoring their program to meet the requirements of those markets. Markets will vary considerably from state to state, among federal jurisdictions, and from one line of insurance to another. Box 13-1 pre-

BOX 13-1

GUIDELINES FOR RESEARCHING THE MARKETPLACE

- Discuss with referral sources how case management fits into their overall company goals. What are they trying to achieve by case management? Is it, for example, medical cost containment, better public relations with subscribers, or returning injured workers to work?
- Identify the lines of authority within the company, especially who is responsible for decision making about case management. Often, it is the chief financial officer (CFO) who decides whether to use case management and from which company to purchase services. Sometimes, the benefits manager and safety/risk manager also are involved. Once the decision to use case management has been made, who is responsible for making referrals and how will potential referrals be identified?
- Research the competition. What are other case management firms offering? Is the referral source using any other firms at present? If so, what kinds of services are being purchased? Are there any issues of dissatisfaction with the current case management providers? This can provide valuable information to help a firm differentiate itself from the competition. Besides obtaining information from referral sources, some other ways of finding out about the competition include:
  - Obtain their marketing materials. This is helpful in identifying their strengths and weaknesses and in developing a unique marketing approach that will be different from theirs.
  - Review their fee structures. Obviously, fees must be in line with the competition, but this aspect needs to be approached cautiously to avoid the appearance of price fixing.
  - Learn about the specialty case management services that are being offered by competitors.
  - Participate in industry associations and professional seminars. Network with the competition.

sents some basic guidelines to follow in researching the marketplace and learning about referral sources.

COMMON EXPECTATIONS OF REFERRAL SOURCES

Often, case management firms make the mistake of assuming that cost savings is the primary or only reason for purchasing services. Although cost savings is an elemental focus, it is not always the only or even the most important factor. In researching the marketplace, case management firms may need to help potential referral sources define what they want. Following are some common expectations of referral sources:

- *Cost savings that are valid and accurately reflect the true effects of case management.* In the past, the dollar savings reported by case management firms was often based on estimates and guesses that may have had little validity. How to accurately measure case management outcomes is covered in depth in Chapter 19. When marketing case management, firms need to be able to present means for assessing the effectiveness of case management in terms of dollar savings.
- *Improved quality of care is a significant factor for many referral sources.* Sometimes (e.g., with Medicaid), assessment of quality of care is an important aspect of case management. Medicaid agencies frequently use case managers to assess whether recipients are receiving appropriate care in various types of **long-term care** facilities. Other types of referral sources expect case managers to refer clients to appropriate providers who meet their needs. Maintenance of quality of care is viewed both as an end in itself and as a component of cost savings because it reduces the chance of complications and other costly factors that may arise.
- *Improved relations with subscribers/employees/unions/claimants.* The positive aspects of case management may help to offset some of the negative connotations that UR may have in the eyes of these individuals. Sometimes, case management firms need to have mechanisms in place to obtain feedback from these individuals to determine whether case management is having a positive impact on employee relations.

DIFFERENTIATING A CASE MANAGEMENT PROGRAM

After the marketplace research has been completed, the focus needs to shift to how a case management program can be differentiated from the competition. Unless a case management firm has something unique to offer, it will seem just like its competitors, and it will not appear to be distinctive enough to address the special needs of the referral source. Box 13-2 describes some effective ways of differentiating a case management program to make it seem especially responsive to the needs of referral sources.

DEVELOPING BROCHURES AND MARKETING MATERIALS

Some of the items that case management firms need to include in their marketing materials have already been mentioned. These include resumes or resume synopses of the qualifications of the staff, sample reports, and references. Case management firms also need to have brochures that explain the history and mission of the company and its service delivery

BOX 13-2

DIFFERENTIATING A CASE MANAGEMENT PROGRAM FROM THE COMPETITION

- *Develop a mechanism (such as file review) and screening criteria for early case identification.* Referral sources know that the potential for cost savings is greater during the early phases of the case when major decisions are being made. (Often, early referral is considered to be contact with a case manager on the first day following an injury.[48]) Having screening criteria that will effectively identify cases with potential to benefit from case management may be beneficial to referral sources. Screening criteria need to be objective and constantly updated based on experience and innovations in both medical practice and managing cases. (See Appendix 1 for examples of screening criteria.)
- *Hire staff with qualifications that address the needs of referral sources.* To show the breadth of skills and expertise of case management staff, have standard resumes and brief resume synopses available for referral sources to review. Inform referral sources that they can choose the case manager they wish to use based on professional background. Case management firms need to decide if they will hire generalists to meet the needs of a varied marketplace or specialist case managers to work in a particular niche.
- *Develop a corporate mission statement* that explains a firm's philosophy of service delivery and, possibly, identifies the marketplace niche it wishes to serve.
- *Develop data reports* for both individual cases and the aggregate from the referral source. Include sample data reports with other marketing materials used. Develop accurate methods for computing cost savings. Be able to communicate the return on investment (ROI) that the referral source can be expected to achieve. (See Chapter 19 on outcomes management for more information on this.)
- *Establish a service delivery model* that can be described in a concrete manner to referral sources to show them how the work will be conducted. Will the service be telephonic or will it include on-site visits? How will cases be handled outside the geographic location of the office? Does the firm hire case managers as employees or independent contractors?
- *Secure the services of physician advisors* in specialty areas that are appropriate to referral sources. This assures the referral source that appropriate physician advisor backup is available when needed.
- *Insurance line specialization.* Does the firm only handle workers' compensation cases or health insurance cases, or does it offer services to all lines of insurance? Are there special teams or units of case managers to handle each line?
- *Establish a fee structure* that is different from the competition. Having the lowest price is not necessarily the best strategy to use, but other, creative pricing structures may convince the referral source that a firm is offering the best deal. Case management firms have traditionally billed hourly on a fee-for-service basis, but some are now using a **capitation** approach or other reimbursement models.
- *Develop procedures for requesting benefits exceptions.* The referral source will want to know how the case manager will obtain permission for benefits exceptions and that their effectiveness, outcome, and cost/benefit effects will be monitored.
- *Determine appropriate procedures for selecting suppliers, resources, and providers* to ensure quality of care.
- *Use references from both referral sources and clients.* Ask other referral sources for permission to use them as references, and be sure to safeguard confidentiality when using letters from clients.

model and fee structure. It may also be beneficial to have samples of screening criteria for case management referrals and samples of tools (such as forms or checklists) that case managers use to match clients to providers and determine justification for benefits exceptions requests.* (See Appendix 1 for examples of screening criteria and forms to use with them.)

Opinions are divided about the value of spending a great deal of money for slick marketing brochures. Some firms are known for their impressive brochures and swear by them. Others believe that it is more important to devote their limited resources to personal attention to referral sources. Some referral sources are impressed by slick brochures because they convey that the firm is large, stable, and financially solvent and has been around for a long time. Other referral sources get a different message—that the firm may be large but somewhat rigid and impersonal and not flexible enough to address special concerns. Some referral sources prefer working with smaller firms because they believe they get more personalized service. These factors must be weighed when a firm is budgeting how much money can be allocated to marketing brochures.

WHO SHOULD PERFORM MARKETING FUNCTIONS?

The answer to this question is that everyone in the firm who has contact with referral sources is marketing. Therefore, staff needs to be trained to be customer oriented in all dealings with referral sources. Staff must be aware of the needs and goals of the referral source and the way they expect to have services delivered. As mentioned earlier, excellent casework is often the best marketing tool available. A good marketing staff may be quite effective in bringing in new business, but a firm will not be able to keep it if it is not providing good casework. Thus staff training and good supervision of casework are essential elements in any marketing program that is based on customer orientation.

Many firms will have special staff who perform marketing functions exclusively. These individuals must not only know how to sell but must also have a high degree of expertise in case management so that they can discuss all aspects of it knowledgeably. It is not enough for them to have a proven but generic track record as sales people. If they are comfortable with selling, case managers often make the best marketers because of their in-depth knowledge of service delivery. They can speak with referral sources in very specific ways about how case management can be beneficial. However, case managers often do not feel comfortable with selling, and caution must be exercised in selecting case managers to be marketers.

Owners or managers of some case management firms often do marketing. This may be effective because of their in-depth knowledge and personal commitment to the firm and because it conveys to referral sources that the firm is interested in customer satisfaction.

Marketing for Case Managers

Some basic guidelines that case managers should keep in mind while working cases and when assisting designated marketing personnel include the following:

*One note of caution in developing marketing materials is that competitors may have access to them. Therefore information that is truly proprietary probably should not be included.

- Remember that every interaction with a customer is a marketing opportunity. This includes routine phone calls on casework, correspondence and reports, and formal marketing visits.
- Remember that what the case manager does will also reflect on the customer because the client tends to view the case manager as an extension of the referral source. For example, if the case manager is extremely insurance oriented and is focused exclusively on cost savings, this attitude will convey to the client that the insurance company wants to save money at the expense of quality of care.
- When making contact with referral sources, listen and probe with the customer about what he or she wants. Do not talk too much. Let the customer talk so that his or her viewpoint becomes evident. Always work within that viewpoint. This is a particularly important point to remember when working with new customers in new lines of business.
- Remember that marketing uses many of the same skills as counseling. Good marketers are also good counselors.
- When working with customers, suggest ideas, get feedback, and modify plans accordingly. Do not just collect data; synthesize information. Show customers your expertise.
- Give the customer information and be available as a resource on both open cases and on cases that have not yet been referred. Encourage the customer to get in the habit of seeking out the advice of a case manager when difficult or nebulous situations arise.
- Always act professionally and use terminology that is appropriate to the situation.
- To learn more about marketing techniques, try shadowing marketing professionals when they make phone calls or visit customers.

The following two dialogues between a customer and a case manager illustrate some of these points:

Poor Interaction

Customer: *I have not heard from you in more than a month on either one of your cases. Do you know how Mr. G. is doing with his return to work?*

Case Manager: *I am not sure what to do with Mr. G. He has not been very cooperative in his follow-through lately. For one thing, I had agreed to request some adaptive equipment so that he can do his job better, but he hasn't returned my calls when I have left messages for him to contact me with information about what he wants. What do you think I should do?*

Better Interaction

Customer: *Thanks for sending me the reports on your cases. I was wondering how Mr. G. is doing on his return to work.*

Case Manager: *Mr. G. has not been very cooperative lately because he did not return my calls when I asked for additional information about the adaptive equipment he requested. Although he has not been good about keeping in touch with me, his employer seems to think he is doing fine in his return to work. Do you want me to continue trying to contact him* *about the job modification? Are there incentives to get him to cooperate with this aspect of his rehabilitation plan? Should I close the case if he does not contact me soon?*

Customer: *Since he has returned to work and is not receiving wage replacement benefits, there are really no incentives to get him to cooperate. Since he seems to be doing all right at work and does not appear to feel any urgency about obtaining the adaptive equipment, I feel that it is time to close the case. If he still wants the adaptive equipment, he can contact me directly.*

Case Manager: *Thank you. I will get the closing report to your office by the end of the week and will send Mr. G. a letter informing him that I am closing his case and that he is to contact you directly if he still wants the equipment.*

It is obvious from the first interaction that the case manager is not focused on maintaining good communication with the customer or exploring the point of view of the customer. The case manager also does not make a very good impression because she only states the facts of the situation and asks the customer to find a solution. In the second interaction, the case manager offers several alternatives from which the customer can choose. The customer is given the opportunity to state her viewpoint, and the case manager reflects back to the customer what she has instructed the case manager to do. In this way, a dialogue has taken place that allows the customer to express what she wants from case management while taking advantage of the case manager's expertise and opinions.

OVERCOMING OBJECTIONS FROM REFERRAL SOURCES

After the marketplace has been researched, a program has been created to differentiate the firm from its competition, and marketing materials have been developed, a formal marketing program can be conducted. In addition to having a thorough knowledge of the case management program and how it can address referral source needs, the person who does marketing also needs to be able to overcome objections from referral sources. Doing a good presentation of the services is not enough; the referral source will not buy unless its objections are effectively addressed. In general, objections are opportunities to present services in an even more positive manner. Here are a number of common objections and ideas for overcoming them:

- *Referrals to case management sometimes result in higher costs rather than cost savings.* Higher costs may result from ill-considered recommendations for benefits exceptions (e.g., outpatient services that may cost more than inpatient treatment) or improper screening of cases for potential to benefit from case management. Sometimes, cases are kept open too long, causing the fees for case management services to offset the medical cost savings. The case management firm needs to have procedures in place to evaluate the ratio of costs to benefits every step of the way.
- *Fear of technical and clinical terminology when communicating with case managers.* Referral sources sometimes think that they will not be able to discuss cases with the case manager in a meaningful way because they will not understand the terminology used. This objection can be overcome by having sample reports that are written in layperson's terms and by not using technical terms during marketing contacts. Case managers need to learn to be sensitive to the educational level of referral source representatives and tailor their language appropriately.

- *Overreferral of cases that have limited capacity to benefit or lack of early referral.* Referral sources want assurance that the case management firm has screening criteria that will identify cases early and will prevent referral of inappropriate cases. If case management is being included with UR services, the UR program will need to have an appropriate screening mechanism that has filters that are neither too narrow nor too broad.
- *Concern that case managers may be too client-advocacy oriented, resulting in higher costs for unnecessary services.* This tends to be a problem with case managers who have a nursing, counseling, or social work background or who have never worked in the private sector. Likewise, case managers may fail to check the benefit plan to determine exclusions and limitations. With good hiring, training, and supervision of case managers, these issues can be minimized.
- *At the opposite extreme, case managers may be too oriented toward saving money at the expense of quality of care.* This problem tends to occur with experienced case managers who may lose sight of the fact that the patient, not the referral source, is the client. Case management tends to be a juggling act of balancing the needs of all parties involved.
- *Lack of comprehensive, timely, accurate reports.* Because reports are the only tangible product of case management, they need to be accurate, well written, informative, and timely. Often, the only aspect of case management that the primary decision maker of a referral source sees are the reports.

Marketing is not a gimmick for short-term gain of market share; it is an ongoing process that touches on all aspects of case management. Firms that are successful are constantly researching the marketplace through networking with the competition, staying abreast of current events in health care reform and legislative changes, and maintaining contact with referral sources. They are constantly incorporating new information into their programs to address specialty niches as they evolve and to further differentiate their services from the competition.

SUGGESTED READINGS

Find, persuade key buyers of CM services; here's how, *Case Management Advisor* 6(4):54-56, 1995.

Garrett MB: Selling and marketing a case management program, *Case Manager* 6(4):59-66, 1995.

How to spread the word about the benefits of case management, *Case Management Advisor* 5(7):94, 99, 1994.

"One-stop shop" approach can help you court self-insured market, *Case Management Advisor* 6(3):29-31, 1995.

Self-promotion offers key to CM survival, *Case Management Advisor* 6(3):32-33, 1995.

References are found at the end of the book.

CHAPTER 14
DEVELOPING A MANAGEMENT PLAN FOR YOUR COMPANY

There is no guaranteed formula for success in case management, but it is generally beneficial to have a management plan when developing a case management program. A management plan is a basic outline of goals, the means for achieving them, outcomes, and time frames that is used to define how a line of business is established and run. Although a management plan will not guarantee success, it is helpful to have one to define how the program will be instituted on a step-by-step basis, who will be responsible for what aspects of it, what criteria will be used to define success, and what long-term and short-term goals are to be achieved. A management plan is most effective when it is written in specific, behaviorally oriented terms that describe what is to be achieved, how it is to be achieved, who is responsible for each step, how success will be measured, and how much time and money can be expended. There are many ways of writing a management plan. Each firm should develop, through experimentation, a format for writing management plans that addresses its own needs.

MARKET RESEARCH

The chapter on marketing preceded this chapter because market research is one of the first steps in developing a management plan for a case management program. Without knowing what the marketplace is like, it would be impossible for a firm to compete with others providing similar services and to develop a program that addresses the needs of potential referral sources. This market research needs to be conducted through interviewing potential referral sources, learning about new developments in health care reform and pertinent legislation, and acquiring knowledge about potential markets (e.g., becoming versed in different lines of insurance).

Market research will help to identify potentially untapped or undermarketed sources of business. Often, the best way to ensure success is to corner a new market, realizing that it may take some time to sell the referral sources in that new market on the idea of case management. Unfortunately, as any marketplace matures, there are fewer and fewer sources of untapped business. However, new markets may be created quite suddenly by any number of legislative, political, and social changes.

The owners and managers of a successful case management firm need to be constantly alert for new opportunities and sources of business in our rapidly changing social and political climate. At all times, firms need to be flexible enough to adapt to the new markets that are created by such changes. Being alert to new business opportunities requires a combination of imagination and creativity.

Market research must include a comparison of competitors to ascertain which ones are apparently the most successful and why. It never hurts to find something that works and imitate it (assuming that it is nonproprietary). Comparing competitors will help to identify new markets that have potential for further development and new services that could be developed to address niches that have not been covered. It will also help firms become different enough from their competitors that they are able to attract the attention of referral sources. No one wants to be just one of a faceless crowd of competitors who are all chasing the same business. The most successful firms always have something unique to offer besides high-quality services.

A management plan needs to not only incorporate how market research will be conducted as the program is being established but also include a plan for ongoing market research that will keep the firm at the top of its field. The management plan must address in very specific ways how information from market research will be evaluated, prioritized, and incorporated into the case management program as it develops. Obviously, not all leads for potential business have the same worth and promise for program development. Some may be quite costly and may not turn a profit for a long time, although the potential for eventual business growth is enormous. Others may be profitable in the short run at a low cost, but their potential may be used up quickly. There is no substitute for holistic, futuristic, proactive thinking in case management because the marketplace changes so rapidly.

ESTABLISHING GOALS

Both long-term and short-term goals can be sifted from the initial market research. Time frames need to be established to assess progress toward goals and to reevaluate goals and set new ones if necessary. Long-term goals generally define the character of the case management company, such as lines of business to establish, anticipated revenue, and referral growth. Short-term goals often delineate some of the tactical steps needed for achieving the long-range goals. Some examples of long-term goals might be to establish a unit to provide case management services to workers' compensation carriers or to write a successful proposal to obtain a contract with a state Medicaid agency. Short-term goals might consist of hiring a case manager with high-risk neonate experience to work on a contract with a specific referral source or opening a second office to serve a new locale.

Once goals are targeted, the firm must determine a step-by-step process for achieving them. A person needs to be designated as the responsible party for achieving each step. In defining each step, the firm must make sure that all of the resources required for achieving it are available.

FINANCIAL PLANNING

A major part of any management plan is the financial section. To keep the firm financially solvent during a period when seed money is being spent but profits have not yet been realized, the firm needs to decide how many resources can be allocated for new program development while still allowing for business as usual in existing programs. Spreadsheets are often helpful in making these calculations.

In general, it is wise to build in cushions because unexpected events and expenses often occur to inflate costs. It is better to have a little in reserve than to overspend, but it is also necessary to spend money to earn money. If inadequate amounts of money are allocated, desired results may not be achieved. This calls for a realistic appraisal of what it will take to achieve a goal. If insufficient funding is available, perhaps the goal is not achievable and needs to be revised. Companies often get into trouble because they waste money on unrealistic projects when they could have secured new business if they had set more modest goals that were within their financial parameters. Be ruthless in evaluating whether the likelihood of success would warrant the anticipated financial expenditure.

Because case management is a service-oriented business, staffing is the greatest expense. Having good staff is also one of the best ways to ensure success through delivering quality services. Having too many staff who are not producing services that can be billed to referral sources is a major financial drain, yet staff will have some nonproductive time at the beginning of the program as it is becoming established. Any firm that is beginning a case management program needs to decide how much nonproductive time can be carried while the program is being launched. Goals must be established regarding productivity and when staff will reach a breakeven point between expenses and revenue generated.

It is hard to give a hard and fast rule on this. Naturally, this will depend on how large the firm is and how much capital it has. Some firms may find that they are too shaky financially to start a case management program because they cannot cover the nonbillable time that will be required to establish it. Their first long-range goal may be to acquire adequate capital or an adequate revenue base to be able to start a program.

PRODUCTIVITY REQUIREMENTS FOR CASE MANAGERS

It is also difficult to say how much productivity (i.e., billable hours or other fee-for-service activities) should be required of each case manager. This depends on the firm, the fees it is able to charge, and the amount of overhead it has. Some firms maintain low overhead by having case managers work out of their homes instead of an office. Other firms have no choice in the matter because their principal referral sources require them to have offices in many locales. Some firms perform work for referral sources who are not so price sensitive; some do business in areas where price competition is quite stiff.

Some referral sources require highly credentialed and experienced case managers who command high salaries and benefits packages; some firms do not have these regulations and can save salary dollars by hiring case managers with lesser qualifications. Some firms control overhead by having case managers work as independent contractors who do not receive benefits and are only paid for billable hours. Often, these arrangements meet both the firm's and the case manager's needs quite effectively because the case manager receives a higher hourly rate and does not have to make a copay for benefits that he or she is already receiving through a spouse's employee benefits program.

Generally, case management programs require full-time case managers to bill between 100 and 150 productive hours per month that can be billed to a referral source. This range tends to be wide because of the differing roles that case managers play in companies. Some firms require case managers to do their own marketing and keep themselves supplied with cases, thus reducing the amount of time they have for billable activities. Lead or supervisory case managers often combine supervision, marketing, and casework. Because case management is so labor intensive, salary and benefits costs need to be balanced carefully with fee structure and anticipated expenses to determine appropriate productivity levels necessary to achieve and maintain profitability.

In addition to productivity, the staffing plan must also address what positions are to be created and what their qualifications are. This will be driven, in part, by the marketplace and the requirements of referral sources. The firm must decide what quality service delivery is and who is likely to be able to provide it adequately. The staffing plan will also address salary ranges, benefits, performance reviews, job descriptions, and lines of authority within the company.

COMPUTER RESOURCES AND OFFICE AUTOMATION

Office automation can be both a cost driver and a means to controlling costs and enhancing productivity. Automation may be costly at the beginning, but if it is balanced against future benefits, it can eliminate some expenses by allowing case managers to work out of their homes and by reducing the number of support staff. Many firms now require case managers to compose their own reports on a word processor, thereby eliminating support staff for this function. Voice mail is used to eliminate or reduce the need for receptionists and telephone operators. Technology also reduces the need for having supervisors in branch offices because supervisors and case managers can communicate by phone, voice mail, and e-mail, and reports can be transmitted to a central office by fax, modem, or the Internet for review.

Computer software designed to meet the needs of case management firms is a recent development that may come more to the forefront in the years to come. Software can be used, for example, to track the way case managers handle certain cases in order to develop guidelines for future use on similar cases.[49]

Some companies have their own custom-designed software, but this is a costly undertaking for small to medium-sized firms. Commercial software systems are available.[50] These systems need to be evaluated carefully in terms of their costs/benefits, especially hidden costs that are involved. There are usually other costs besides the hardware, software, and initial installation, including time for creating support files, staff training time to learn the system, possible downtime if the system crashes while "bugs" are being worked out of it, ongoing monthly charges, and possible need for hiring a programmer or consultant to customize the software.

If the firm is also offering UR, screening criteria for case management can be incorporated into review software, thereby producing an instant, objective screening of all certification cases that might have potential to benefit. Firms that do not provide UR may also be able to have custom software programs developed that will provide quick screening of cases, thereby saving staff time. Of course, systems of this nature tend to be costly, but the savings in terms of staff time and the benefit of having something different from the competition may outweigh the expense. All of these considerations need to weighed carefully in any decision making.[51]

The management plan will also cover the establishment of the case management office or unit and how it is to be run. Will case managers work in offices or at home? What kinds of equipment and supplies are needed? How will the office be laid out? (More information on this is contained in Chapter 15.)

The management plan may also incorporate long-range plans for growth and the opening of new markets. What additional services can be added later to enhance existing services? What other markets have potential but will require more than the current level of capitalization? **Quality assurance (QA)** is another important issue. To retain referral sources and secure repeat business, the quality of case management services needs to be assessed on an ongoing basis. Who will do this, and what tools will they use to aid them? Referral sources will not continue to do business with a firm if they are not receiving quality services. Thus each firm also needs to develop the ability to assess the effectiveness of its case management program and present that information to the referral source in the form of outcome reports. (More about quality assurance and outcomes management in later chapters.)

Writing and executing a management plan needs to be a joint effort among all staff involved. Marketing staff need to perform the market research and to make recommendations based on it. Owners and managers need to weigh potential sources of business against the cost of developing them or of establishing a case management program at all. Owners, managers, and supervisors need to establish productivity goals and to discuss how they will be achieved (e.g., whether incentives will be used) and time frames for installation.

If the firm hopes to secure contracts with referral sources, this needs to be included in the management plan. These contracts often represent major sources of business and require an enormous amount of preparation to obtain. Government contracts, especially, usually require a written response to a Request for Proposal (RFP). These proposals sometimes number in the hundreds of pages and require a formal oral interview complete with audiovisual aids. To be competitive in responding to some of these RFPs, it may be necessary to invest money in developing new programs and to secure the assistance of outside consultants, such as grant writers. Special attention needs to be paid to budgetary considerations when considering whether to respond to an RFP. Because of economies of scale, the nature of the competition, and required startup costs, some RFPs may not be profitable. Although most of them have escape clauses for the relief of firms who may be in over their heads, backing out of a contract may be too costly in terms of loss of reputation and goodwill.

Once a management plan has been written, it should be reevaluated on a regular basis to assess progress and make updates as necessary. A management plan is not a static process; to be effective, it must evolve constantly. Sometimes, management plans that are not working need to be scrapped entirely, and new ones have to be developed. A firm's management plan forms the foundation of its program and must always be adaptable to changes as they occur.

SUGGESTED READINGS

Maeling JA, Badger K: Information systems tools available to the case manager, *Nursing Case Management* 1(1):35-40, 1996.

Computerization: don't byte off more bits than you can chew, *Case Management Advisor* 6(2):17-21, 1995.

Software takes big byte out of CM workload, *Case Management Advisor* 6(7):93-94, 99-101, 1995.

Software: supports for field CM efforts, *Case Management Advisor* 7(1):15-16, 1996.

References are found at the end of the book.

CHAPTER 15
THE CASE MANAGEMENT OFFICE OR UNIT

A well-run office is essential to any case management program. A case management program will need to be incorporated into the existing structure of a firm that develops it. Although every case management office and firm are different, this chapter covers some basic issues that need to be addressed in order to provide quality services in an efficient manner that will enable the firm to be profitable. These guidelines should be evaluated and adapted to fit the needs of individual firms.

STAFFING AND ORGANIZATION

Case managers need to be supervised by someone who is qualified to give them guidance. Ideally, this will be someone with a case management background. In small firms that have only one or two case managers, the supervisor may not be a case manager but still must be someone who is familiar enough with the issues of case management to provide guidance. Small firms may designate one case manager as the lead. This person will carry a caseload but will also perform the supervisory functions of reviewing files and reports and staffing cases with case managers.

Supervisors should be located in the same office as case managers or should be readily accessible at all times by phone, voice mail, or e-mail. Case management is, by its very nature, a job filled with complex issues and tough decisions. Having supervisory help available will provide new knowledge and other ways of thinking and handling the ambiguous situations that always seem to arise. Particularly for new case managers, supervision is a learning experience to acquire new knowledge, expertise with different medical conditions, and a different point of view. Even for case managers who have been in the business for many years, supervision affords an opportunity for learning in a field in which knowledge expands exponentially.

The supervisor needs to meet with case managers on a regular basis to discuss cases and provide information and suggestions on how to work cases more effectively. The supervisor must review all cases periodically to ensure that they are being worked properly and that the reporting and recommendations are appropriate. Some supervisory functions, such as reviewing invoices, may be performed by the case management supervisor or someone who is higher up in the organization.

Marketing responsibilities need to be delegated to either designated marketing staff, case managers, supervisors, or management staff within the firm.

JOB DESCRIPTIONS

The most essential ingredient, however, in staffing the case management unit is to develop accurate and complete descriptions of each job. It has been said that "a job description should include all areas of case management function based on CMSA's *Standards of Practice for Case Management*."[52] Job descriptions need to clearly describe everyone's roles and the amount of time that is to be devoted to them. It is important to note that a comprehensive job description is the basis for qualification for the CCM examination.

The job description should begin with a position summary and go on to describe the duties and responsibilities of the entire case management department, including who will provide direct supervision. Duties and responsibilities are an important component of the job description. Basing these on CMSA's *Standards of Practice for Case Management* will help direct and focus both the responsibilities of the position and the focus of the case management department as a whole. At a minimum, the following duties and responsibilities should be included:

- Identify and screen potential cases for case management
- Monitor and manage the care plan
- Communicate with all involved participants
- Advocate

The job description should emphasize likely outcomes, scope of influence, and learning as a fundamental part of the job and an ongoing condition of employment.

PERFORMANCE EVALUATIONS

Performance objectives need to be developed for each staff member, and a system for periodic performance review needs to be in place. The performance evaluation not only assesses past performance but also helps set goals and serves as a developmental tool. Guidelines to positive performance evaluations include:

- Make the evaluation part of an ongoing process rather than an isolated event.
- Keep notes of performance observations.
- Focus on the relationship, not the paper form.
- Schedule two meetings to complete the evaluation. During the first meeting, review your assessment and the reasons for your opinions with the CM, allowing time for him or her to participate in the process and giving the supervisor an opportunity to finetune the information. The second, much shorter meeting will complete the final process.

SUPPORT STAFF

How much support staff will be needed will depend on office automation and office systems used. Using voice mail and having case managers word process their own letters and reports substantially decreases the amount of support staff needed. In general, it is helpful to have support staff designated for the case management program rather than just having work go into a general typing pool. Designated support staff are able to maintain a higher level of knowledge about medical terminology and case management and are, thus, able to be more accurate and productive.

OFFICE SYSTEMS

Office systems have to be developed to handle word processing, supervision of reports, maintenance of records and files, invoicing, and payroll. Many firms either link billable hours into payroll or have very specific billable hours expectations for case managers. Firms that only pay case managers for billable hours need accurate billing information on a weekly basis in order to generate payroll. Some firms use staff productivity measures for budgeting and projecting profitability or to award monthly, quarterly, or yearly bonuses based on billable hours. To address these needs, many firms have daily time sheets that case managers complete as they perform billable activities on cases. Sometimes, these time sheets are automated into computer networks. Usually, time sheets are turned in daily or faxed or transmitted to a central location.

In addition to the case manager's name and the date, time sheets generally record the name of the client, the type of activity or expense, and the amount of time to be billed, which is recorded in tenths of an hour. This type of system records not only the number of hours billed by the case manager but also the hours and expenses to be billed to the referral source.

This billable hours system is effective for fee-for-service work, but other systems have to be developed for capitation billing or flat rate billing. These billing alternatives generally require a software program that monitors the expense of doing business in relationship to the revenues generated. Capitation and flat rate billing can be based on billable hours requirements for case managers, but the number of hours expended per referral source has to be monitored carefully to ensure that casework is being conducted in an efficient manner and referral sources are not being given more services than they are paying for.

Maintenance of records and files involves both individual cases and the aggregate of cases from each referral source. Referral sources want to know whether positive outcomes are being produced on cases. This requires a system (preferably automated) that tracks the pertinent factors on which the referral source wants information and may include average length of time cases are open, dollars saved as a result of case management, dollars spent on case management, net savings, and outcomes for the client (e.g., return to independent living, return to work, long-term residential care). Some outcome measurements also track quality of care issues. Some automated systems track this automatically when the case manager or supervisor fills in key data elements as the case is closed. Other systems require the case manager to complete a form that is turned in for data entry.

Outcome statistics need to be kept on each referral source and are used to generate reports to show the effectiveness of the case management program. These reports are often required quarterly or yearly by the referral source.

Most firms use case files that may be automated or kept in file folders. Case files generally contain all referral information reports, medical records, other records, invoices, correspondence, case notes, and other pertinent information obtained in the course of working cases. Sometimes, four-part or six-part folders are used to organize information by category. Some firms have only one file folder, whereas others maintain a working file that is kept by the case manager and a master file that is kept in the office at all times. The advantage of having duplicate files is that there is a backup in case of a loss, and supervisors, administrators, and accounting staff can consult file information when necessary if the case manager has the file out of the office.

Systems have to be developed to ensure that all paperwork is copied and routed to the appropriate file and that files are kept in an orderly fashion, because some cases may be subject to periodic audit by the referral source. When cases are closed, files have to be archived for a number of years depending on jurisdiction. Good file maintenance also requires that procedures be followed to ensure client confidentiality.

Records of other activities besides casework and referral source databases also have to be kept. Good record keeping is an essential part of any marketing program in order to be well organized and systematic in opening new avenues of business. These records must include which referral sources have been contacted by whom for what purpose with what outcome. Overall outcome statistics should be kept for the company as a whole. These are often very valuable as marketing tools to show the superiority of one's services when compared with the competition. If the firm contracts with specific referral sources, especially government agencies, additional records with very exact specifications may be required.

Whether reports and correspondence are word processed by case managers or support staff, systems have to be in place to ensure that they are supervised as appropriate. With some automated systems, the case manager or support staff can have the supervisor review the material on computer and make changes as necessary. Supervisors in other firms review and make changes to hard copies. Review of invoices against case notes requires the supervisor to either have a hard copy of the case notes or have access to case notes that are kept on computer.

DATA SYSTEMS AND OFFICE AUTOMATION

All of these considerations point to the necessity of having good computer support when developing any type of office system for case management. Although a few firms still get by with a minimum of automation, good computer support is becoming more and more of a necessity to maintain competitiveness in this business.

Choosing appropriate software for a case management program is a difficult and confusing job that may require the services of a consultant. Custom systems are available, and commercial products may be customized to meet the needs of individual firms. In general, if a great deal of customization is needed, the software product is probably not appropriate.[53] Whatever software is used must have the flexibility to meet reporting capabilities required by the firm and referral sources.

To choose software, it is necessary to know what you want the software to do and to define your goals for the software. Developing a list of desired features is often effective, especially if you prioritize what you want and define areas of possible compromise. A database system consultant or in-house staff person can assist in the development of a selection criteria list. Some other things that need to be evaluated include how user-friendly and flexible the system is. Will it be possible to integrate the software with the current operating system and databases? Are the user manuals clear and easy to use?

The selection process will generally take 6 to 9 months. After a number of products have been reviewed, the list should be narrowed to three or four vendors who will be evaluated in detail. Often, the best way to evaluate a system is to contact other case management firms who are using it and interview them carefully about their experiences with it. Demonstrations of software are also a must, but time can be saved by doing the demonstration over a modem.

Once a system has been selected, the implementation process will be an ongoing project. Most likely, a permanent, full-time staff member will need to be assigned to handle staff training and system support and maintenance issues.

ADMINISTERING CONTRACTS

Extensive systems often need to be developed for administering contracts, especially those with government agencies. Frequently, these systems need to be already in place and open for inspection for consideration. Generally, contract administration requires the ability to track program statistics, to be open for periodic audits, to organize and maintain files in an orderly manner, to have systems for safeguarding data and confidentiality, to have fail-safes to ensure adherence to time lines, to be able to transmit data to the referral source electronically or interactively, and, sometimes, to be able to track statistics on health care providers and quality of care. Before bidding on any contracts or RFPs, firms need to assess their internal systems and upgrade them as necessary.

OFFICE SPACE, FURNITURE, AND EQUIPMENT

In many respects, case management does not require much startup money to be operational because it does not require much office space and equipment if case managers work mostly out of their homes. However, with the advent of automation, a great deal of money can be spent on computers, software, and other labor-saving devices. In drawing up a management plan (see Chapter 14), each firm needs to carefully consider the cost/benefit of the options that are available and choose the ones that are the most viable given the nature of the referral sources with which it expects to be working.

As electronic communication becomes more and more prevalent, case managers will need to be connected to the outside world via the Internet and have ready access to fax and e-mail for communications. The ability of the case manager to communicate electronically will be essential whether the case manager is working out of a home or an office environment. It is beyond the scope of this book to discuss specific systems available. Suggested readings at the end of this chapter will be helpful for more details about available electronic systems.

Regardless of what electronic systems case managers may have, they will also need a well-stocked library of basic resources. These include a medical dictionary, information about customers' insurance plans, prescription drug handbooks, and other textbooks related to medicine, nursing, and rehabilitation. A suggested list of resources is included in Chapter 12.

SUGGESTED READINGS

Computerization: don't byte off more bits than you can chew, *Case Management Advisor* 6(2):17-21, 1995.

Maeling JA, Badger K: Information systems tools available to the case manager, *Nursing Case Management* 1(1):35-40, 1996.

Software takes big byte out of CM workload, *Case Management Advisor* 6(7):93-94, 99-101, 1995.

Van Genderen A: How to develop and manage a case management department, *J Care Management* 2(4):30-41, 1996.

References are found at the end of the book.

CHAPTER 16
HIRING, TRAINING, AND SUPERVISION OF CASE MANAGERS

The subject of case manager qualifications was discussed in Chapter 3. Basically, case managers need to meet the requirements of referral sources in terms of education, experience, and certifications. Their qualifications also need to be congruent with the type of case management program being offered. (Refer to Chapter 3 for more complete information on this.)

RECRUITING AND HIRING CASE MANAGERS

It has been found that because "the single most critical variable in the success of case management practice is the skill of the case manager,"[54] good recruiting and hiring are of paramount importance.

There are many different approaches that can be used to recruit qualified case managers. In some areas of the country, there is still a nursing shortage, which makes it difficult to recruit nurse case managers. This problem has eased up considerably in recent years in some parts of the country as a result of health care reform, but recruitment still tends to be difficult because merely having a nursing background does not adequately prepare a nurse to do case management.

One of the most effective recruitment techniques tends to be networking or word-of-mouth. This technique relies on the personal contacts of the person doing the hiring. The main advantage to networking is that it tends to recruit individuals who already have a good reputation among their peers. Usually, this is less risky than hiring someone who is not personally known to anyone who knows the recruiter. Even the best efforts at checking references sometimes prove to be fruitless because employers are increasingly concerned about litigation and often will not provide much meaningful information about former workers.

Another effective recruiting method is to contact professional associations. Professional associations with state or local chapters, such as CMSA or NARPPS, often have newsletters that will accept want ads. Making announcements and doing informal networking at professional meetings and workshops is often productive as well.

Recruiting through newspaper want ads requires a well-written ad. Ads should represent the job and the firm accurately and should also make the work seem interesting and appealing. The ad should indicate that the job requires independent work, creativity, ingenuity, a good business sense, knowledge of insurance, and ability to market.

One common recruitment approach that is not recommended is visiting colleges and universities. Ordinarily, individuals who are just out of school do not have the experience, business sense, and breadth of knowledge to be effective as case managers. Case management is not an entry-level occupation.

Resumes are screened to ascertain whether candidates have the basic education and experience required for the job. Following are types of general experience that often are beneficial:

- Rehabilitation
- Public health nursing
- Utilization review
- Orthopedics (especially for workers' compensation)
- Psychiatric nursing (counseling skills)
- Strong clinical experience in related areas
- A background in insurance
- Quality assurance
- Marketing

Interviews with candidates should cover all the pertinent issues described in Chapter 3. They should also be directed at providing information on case management and finding out whether the individual is temperamentally suited to this kind of work. Some individuals with nursing, social work, or counseling backgrounds do not adjust well to case management because they are too client-advocacy oriented. These individuals often express frustration because they must work within the constraints of an insurance system that may not be responsible for providing some of the things clients urgently need.

Other would-be case managers do not adjust well to the unstructured nature of case management, especially having to function as a generalist and acquire information as the case is worked. Case management requires individuals to be self-starters who can work independently and have well-developed skills at managing their time and setting priorities. Still other candidates experience difficulty with having to account for all of their time (i.e., billable hours).

Case managers must be emotionally mature and assertive in their dealings with others. Emotional maturity may be present at any age and is evidenced by responsive answers to questions, good listening skills, interest in others, and the ability to avoid interjecting personal biases into situations. In general, as much time should be devoted to interviewing candidates about their temperamental qualities as their education and experience.

Other factors that can be assessed during job interviews include the following:

- Written and oral communication skills—ask the candidate to bring a writing sample to the interview
- Time management, flexibility, and autonomy[55]
- A professional appearance and demeanor
- Ability to handle ethical dilemmas—pose some hypothetical situations and ask the candidate to respond to them
- Ability to address issues related to cost effectiveness—pose hypothetical situations
- Ability to synthesize information and make recommendations

Because hiring good case managers is crucial to the success of any case management program, plenty of time should be devoted to the hiring process. It is often valuable to have candidates come in for more than one interview. References should be checked carefully. Because employers are concerned about litigation, often the best references are obtained through networking. Generally, it is not beneficial to contact the references that are listed by the candidate, as most job seekers are savvy enough to list references who will give only positive information about them.

During the initial interview, it is essential to identify personal issues that can affect the candidate's ability to work effectively as a case manager. For example, candidates who are likely to become frustrated working within the constraints of an insurance system or who are trying to meet their own needs through a case management role do not become successful case managers. Individuals who lack a sense of patient advocacy or commitment to assess and problem solve proactively find it impossible to develop a collaborative approach to case management. They are often ineffective and adversarial in their dealings with clients and providers.

Open-ended questions during the interview can be very helpful in identifying the appropriate candidate for the position. These types of questions can help determine if the candidate has the temperament and skills to work effectively as a case manager. Examples of questions of this type include the following:

- What is your motivation in pursuing a position in case management?
- What is your perception of the case manager's job functions?
- What impact could you make as a case manager in this position?
- Describe how you have dealt with difficult or conflicting situations. Give examples.
- Clinically, have you ever made a mistake? If so, what did you do about it, and what did you learn from it?
- Describe how you manage your time and set priorities.

TRAINING NEW CASE MANAGERS

The chapters in this book (especially Part I and Part II) can be used as a basic outline for training case managers. It is helpful to have new case managers read this book and *The Case Manager's Handbook* by Catherine M. Mullahy.[56] However, there is no substitute for going over the basics of case management in a group setting that allows for discussion and exploration of issues.

Each case management firm must develop a training program that will address its needs and the requirements of its major referral sources. Training programs are most effective if they follow a prescribed outline and include handouts and group or individual exercises. In addition to the subjects covered in Parts I and II of this book, a training outline should include the following:

- A module on marketing because every contact with a referral source is a potential marketing opportunity. All case managers should know the general principles of marketing even if they will not be functioning in a designated marketing role.
- Information on the history, mission, and philosophy of the firm.
- The organizational structure of the firm, including staff, office procedures, fee schedule, billing, quality assurance, and performance expectations.

- The history, mission, and philosophy of major referral sources and information on their expectations of case management and how to work with them effectively.

The most effective training programs are geared to the education and previous job experience of the new case managers. A firm's basic training and orientation program can be adapted to include more information for inexperienced case managers and can be condensed for case managers with previous experience.

Training and orientation usually involve some classroom instruction. They may also involve a performance phase, which is described below. Ordinarily, training and orientation will last from a couple of days to a week or longer, depending on the experience level of the case manager. At the end of the orientation phase, it is helpful to have a self-administered, open-book test to help the case manager and supervisor assess what the case manager has learned and what still needs improvement. (An example of this type of test is found in Appendix 4.)

It is often helpful for the supervisor or trainer to accompany case managers who are completely inexperienced on their first visits to the client and the attending physician. This allows the supervisor to address any problem areas and gives the case manager the opportunity to ask questions that might not have been apparent during the classroom part of the orientation. Supervisors may find it useful to listen in on phone calls during the case manager's first few days working cases.

CONTINUING EDUCATION

Most firms provide some form of inservice training to case managers on an ongoing basis or will pay for case managers to attend some workshops and conferences every year. Case managers often must obtain continuing education credits to maintain state RN licensure, CCM or CDMS certification, and other credentials. Most firms require or encourage case managers to maintain and upgrade their credentials. Many firms will provide some funding toward this end.

SUPERVISION OF CASE MANAGERS

Good supervision of case managers is a major component in quality assurance of casework, and case management firms should develop formal service standards against which all case management work is measured. It has been observed that "these service standards should be general ones specifying time lines and which services are delivered during the different phases of the case management process. These phases usually consist of assessment, treatment plan development and treatment plan execution and monitoring."[57]

Each case manager needs to have someone who is designated as his or her supervisor. The supervisor needs to meet with the case manager on a regular basis to review cases and provide information and suggestions on how to work cases more effectively. All case files need to be reviewed periodically by the supervisor to ensure that they are being worked properly, billing is appropriate, and time lines are being met. Supervisors usually document file reviews in case files. It is customary in most case management firms for the supervisor to also read each report before it is mailed, faxed, or transmitted to the referral source. The written correspondence of new case managers sometimes is read. Many firms have a policy of supervisory review of all invoices to ensure that billing is accurate and all activities are documented in case notes.

Box 16-1 presents a list of issues and concerns to which supervisors should attend when supervising reports and case files for quality assurance.

Although these guidelines are generally useful, supervising case management tends to be an art rather than a science. Supervisors must tailor their approach to the individual expertise of the case manager and the case at hand. Supervision requires an enormous amount of creativity, problem-solving ability, and knowledge about where to look for answers. Essentially, the case management supervisor is an information broker who assists the case manager in acquiring the knowledge and information to work the case effectively.

Another role of the supervisor of case managers is to assign cases to the appropriate case manager. The ability to do this effectively is gained by becoming thoroughly familiar with

BOX 16-1

QA POINTS TO ADDRESS WHEN SUPERVISING REPORTS AND CASE FILES

- Have the client's assets and limitations been clearly identified? Are there areas of concern that need further evaluation? Is further assessment warranted? Does it appear that there are complicating conditions, such as substance abuse, impeding progress?
- Have realistic objectives been established, and have they been described in terms of who, what, where, when, why, and how much?
- Do objectives and recommendations appear to be cost effective?
- Have alternatives been thoroughly explored to identify and compare options to maintain quality of care and obtain the best prices? Have price negotiations taken place with providers? Could the client be safely moved to a less costly treatment setting? Can family members be trained as caregivers?
- Does case activity, as reflected in case notes, correspond with the billing? Are amounts billed appropriate in relationship to the activity performed? For example, billing an hour for a phone call would look suspicious.
- Is case management saving more money than it is costing? Is case closure warranted at this time?
- Are services being delivered in a timely manner?
- Would benefits exceptions be warranted? If so, have different options been costed out and compared?
- Is the client ready to return to work? What steps need to be taken for the client to return to work?
- Would the services of a physician advisor be beneficial? Are board-certified physicians being used for IMEs and other referrals? Are appropriate treatment providers being used?
- Are there any ethical issues that need to be addressed? Is the case manager maintaining professional objectivity?
- Is the file well organized? Is anything missing?
- Is the case being worked actively, or is the case manager merely performing passive monitoring activities?
- Is the confidentiality of the case being maintained?

the strengths and weaknesses of the case managers being supervised, as well as the needs of the types of cases that are referred. Part of assigning cases is ensuring that case managers have enough cases to meet their billable hour quotas but not so many that there are not enough hours in the regular work day to give proper attention to each case. The appropriate size caseload will vary according to whether catastrophic cases are being handled and how many cases are telephonic. This can range from as few as 10 cases to as many as 60 if the caseload is exclusively telephonic.[58]

SUGGESTED READINGS

Case management caseloads: how much is too much? *Case Management Advisor* 6(5):61-64, 1995.

Hodge M: Supervising case managers, *Psychosocial Rehabilitation J* 12(3):51-59, 1989.

Lowery SL: Hiring right—qualifications for the successful case manager, *Case Manager* 3(4):66-68, 70-71, 73-74, 1992.

Meeks K, Balfour J, Merritt R, Siefker JM: Guidelines for supervision of medical case management, *NARPPS J News* 6(6):251-255, 1991.

Shipske G: An overview of case management supervision, *Caring* 6(12):5-10, 1987.

Van Genderen A: How to develop and manage a case management department, *J Care Management* 2(4): 30-41, 1996.

References are found at the end of the book.

CHAPTER 17

RISK MANAGEMENT IN CASE MANAGEMENT

To manage the risk inherent in case management, a firm's case management program must be clearly defined and described for all stakeholders involved (i.e., clients, physicians, referral sources). All of the parties involved need to understand the role of case management and the duties and responsibilities of the case manager (saving money for the referral source, obtaining necessary services for the client, and monitoring the performance of providers/vendors). The case manager will have to balance all of these goals and expectations. Honest and responsive answers to inquiries about the role and goals of case management need to be promptly delivered, so the inquiring party understands what case management can and cannot do, as well as what the process typically involves. Misunderstanding of the case manager's role tends to be a major factor in the rising incidence of legal actions against case managers.[59]

ELEMENTS OF A GOOD CASE MANAGEMENT PROGRAM

An outstanding case management program begins with hiring well-qualified candidates for the case management positions. Verification of employment, background, and licensure/certification needs to occur to secure skilled professionals. These processes of verification of licensure and certification need to continue throughout the case manager's employment at the firm to ensure that there are no legal or ethical issues that affect the case manager's practice.

Once case managers have been hired, the firm needs to have a defined training program in place, including policies and procedures about various aspects of case management. A check list of items to be covered in training could be developed to assess the case manager's progress through the orientation process. A preceptorship, or buddy, system could be developed where new case managers are assigned to seasoned case managers to enhance their learning through observation of actual practice and application of the policies and procedures learned through the orientation program.

Initially, a new case manager may require intensive supervision and guidance, especially in regard to the *Standards of Practice for Case Management.*[60] Weak areas will depend on the individual case manager, but they could involve interviewing skills, report writing, and recommendation development. Close scrutiny by a supervisor of such areas as appropriateness of billable hours, compliance with reporting time frames, appropriateness of recommendations, and thoroughness of report writing will help to ensure the integrity of the case management program. (See Chapter 18 on internal quality control for further elaboration.)

Formal and informal feedback from clients/families and referral sources is also a way to determine if the case management program is successful in meeting expectations and functioning within defined parameters. However, it should be noted that case managers can be well liked by clients or referral sources, but they may fail to adhere to certain standards, such as report writing. For example, a case manager may keep the referral source well informed on the case through frequent telephone contacts, and the referral source may be pleased with the resulting close relationship. Yet the case manager may fail to write timely reports and generate invoicing for the firm.

Case managers need to understand the needs and specifications of each referral source. Account/referral source specific instructions may need to be developed to assist the case manager in understanding his or her role. The case manager may also need to have a basic understanding of the insurance coverage and benefit plan to properly work the assigned cases. Specifically, the case manager needs to know what authority he or she has when it comes to authorizing certain health care services, especially when benefits exceptions are involved. If a case manager becomes overzealous in assisting clients, he or she may imply that certain health care services are authorized or approved for payment when, in reality, the referral source has requested to review and approve such situations. Case managers also need to be aware that "given the cost of health care services today, payment decisions are treatment decisions."[61] Thus a case manager who recommends that a payer withhold payment for a recommended treatment may be opening herself or himself up to liability if the patient suffers significant adverse effects. These areas need to be covered in case manager training in order to avoid confusion and the resulting consequences.

More and more, case management involves provider/vendor negotiations and client placement. Inherent in this is the potential for case managers to receive financial incentives for channeling or directing patients to certain facilities. Case management firms may also receive nonfinancial incentives from certain providers, such as inhouse staff training. It is critical for firms to communicate to their case managers the desired relationships with providers/vendors, including clear boundaries on accepted, professional behavior. Any breach of this policy could seriously jeopardize client relations and referral sources, and there may be legal implications. In addition, case managers may have the ability to recommend, authorize, or select certain providers/vendors for their clients, but this power should not go to their heads. In other words, case managers need to understand that they still need to treat all parties in the case management process professionally and with respect to retain the necessary integrity.

Access and availability of necessary resources to conduct professional case management is the responsibility of the case management firm. Since the job of the case manager requires a variety of knowledge, the firm should supply information on how to access necessary resources. A resource file could be established as well as an address database for the case manager to use when selecting necessary services for clients. In particular, the case management firm should make medical/health care resources available for case managers who may need assistance in dealing with a specific condition or illness. This could be supplied through medical literature, physician advisors, supervisors, or other case managers who have specific clinical expertise. In any event, the case manager needs to understand how he or she can obtain assistance in dealing with unfamiliar medical issues.

POLICIES AND PROCEDURES FOR CASE MANAGEMENT

To better manage the risks involved in case management, the policies and procedures for case management should include the items listed below:

- *Confidentiality regulations, restrictions, rights, and responsibilities may vary from jurisdiction to jurisdiction.* Certain regulations may apply if the case involves a Medicaid beneficiary, and different regulations may apply if the case involves an injured worker covered under workers' compensation. Case managers need to understand the necessity and function of release forms from clients or their legal representative. Clients also need to understand that the information shared during an interview with a case manager will most likely be communicated to the referral source. This refers to the recommendation made earlier that case managers should be clear and open about their role.
- *Policies and procedures for the reporting of "incidents" such as car wrecks during the course of casework or negative encounters with clients or referral sources need to be established.* Incidents may also involve unreasonable, unethical, or illegal requests from referral sources, physicians, vendors, providers, or clients. Case managers need to understand the need for supervisors or managers to be informed of such sensitive situations as soon as possible so that appropriate actions can be implemented.
- *A policy and procedure for reporting suspected child/elder abuse should be in place to assist case managers in reporting such incidents.* State and federal law may need to be researched to determine the legal requirements for such situations. Since case management may be delivered in different ways, there may need to be one policy and procedure for telephonic case management and another for on-site case management. If the case managers are licensed health care professionals (e.g., RNs), there may be specific reporting requirements for these situations.
- *Exposure to communicable diseases may occur if the service delivery model for a case management firm includes on-site visits.* A policy and procedure may need to be in place to provide direction for case managers who may be exposed to such situations during on-site visits. Universal precautions could define how case managers should function when exposed to communicable diseases during the course of their casework.
- *Case managers may also encounter potentially dangerous or violent situations during on-site visits.* Clients or family members may have lethal weapons, engage in illegal drug use, consume alcohol, or engage in abusive behavior. Case managers need to know what their rights and responsibilities are under such circumstances. Same-gender case managers may need to be assigned to certain clients if there are legitimate concerns regarding the client, or two people in attendance during an on-site visit could also be helpful.
- *Case managers may encounter clients who are potentially suicidal.* There are state and possibly federal regulations and laws that govern the reporting of such incidents. Licensed health care professionals may have explicit responsibilities regarding the reporting of such situations. Case managers need to understand the process of detecting, confirming, and reporting suicidal cases to the proper legal and medical authorities, as well as to management.

- *Other medical issues may arise during casework that may need to be addressed by the firm.* These may include guidelines on how to advise a client who, for example, is pregnant and has learned that there are serious genetic defects with the fetus/unborn baby and is considering an abortion. Another situation might be a client who is terminally ill and is wanting to exercise a right-to-die option. These are very difficult situations and may require additional professional, medical, risk management, and ethical consultation.

These examples are meant to provide some strategies and ideas on how to better manage the inherent risk in conducting case management activities. There have been an increasing number of lawsuits brought against case managers and their firms, especially as case management grows in its use. These risk management issues, as well as the legal and ethical issues described elsewhere, need to be addressed by a case management firm in order to continue to offer an integrity program full of legal problems.

SUGGESTED READINGS

Banja JD: Ethics, conflicts of interest. I. *Case Manager* 2(4):24, 26, 1991.

Banja JD: Ethics, conflicts of interest. II. *Case Manager* 3(1):20, 22, 1992.

Case Management Society of America: *CMSA, Case Management Society of America, standards of practice,* Little Rock, Ark, 1995, Author.

Clear, complete communication helps CMs safely navigate legal minefields, *Case Management Advisor* 8(3):41-44, 1997.

Hogue EE: Are case managers liable? *J Care Management* 1(2):35-38, 1995.

References are found at the end of the book.

CHAPTER 18
INTERNAL QUALITY CONTROL

Maintenance of high-quality casework is essential to the success of any case management program because it will be reflected in high referral source satisfaction and increased referrals of cases. It has been noted that "quality improvement in . . . case management is [also] necessary to protect consumers and to enhance the clinical practice of case management."[62] As mentioned in other chapters, casework performance standards need to be developed by each case management firm according to guidelines and expectations of referral sources. These standards are used to form the basis for any internal quality control program.

Most internal quality control programs involve the periodic review of all case files by the supervisor to determine if the casework performance standards are being met. These reviews are generally made about once a month while the case is open. Sometimes, cases are reviewed in their entirety when they are closed to determine the reasons for unusual circumstances, such as overly high billing, unfavorable outcomes, or referral source dissatisfaction.

To be time efficient on monthly file reviews, the supervisor ordinarily does not review the whole case but only case notes, reports, and other information that have been produced since the last review. If the case is open a long time, it may be reviewed in its entirety about every 3 months to ensure that it is moving along in an efficient manner. Sometimes, managers or owners periodically review a certain percentage of open and closed cases as a check on the quality of the supervisor's work and the overall case management program.

As well as ensuring that casework is being conducted appropriately and referral sources are satisfied, file review also acts as a supervisory tool. Because much of case management is not subject to direct observation, regular review of files is one of the few ways that a supervisor has of checking on the quality of the services being delivered. Thus, file review is a component of the ongoing performance review of case managers. It can be used to identify areas of strength that can be capitalized on when assigning cases, and it helps to identify weak areas that can be improved through training and appropriate performance planning and objectives. Supervisors can use these reviews when staffing cases with case managers to problem solve difficult situations that arise and to assist new case managers at becoming more proficient.

CHECKLISTS AS A FILE REVIEW TOOL

Most firms use checklists based on their performance standards as a tool in reviewing files. These checklists are kept in the file folder and serve as a reminder that certain things need to be addressed as the case is worked. They also serve as documentation of file review and act as a report card for the supervisor as well as the case manager. They are also helpful if there is a change of case manager or supervisor. By merely glancing at them, a person who is new to the case can see if certain things have been accomplished and what needs to take place in the near future. Checklists are also valuable when working with referral sources that have unusual or highly detailed requirements. Individual checklists can be developed for these accounts to assist the case manager and supervisor in attending to the myriad of details required by some referral sources.

Checklists are partly for the documentation of factual information (such as when the last report was written), but they also address more global issues, such as whether recommendations are appropriate. A word of caution is in order, however. Although checklists are helpful, they tend to focus on details, sometimes to the exclusion of the big picture. The supervisor must still look at the case in its entirety to determine whether its overall direction is appropriate and whether case management is accomplishing anything worthwhile. Box 18-1 presents some of the critical elements to include on internal quality control checklists.[63]

FLOWCHARTS

As well as checklists, flowcharting is sometimes helpful in assessing and maintaining quality in case management services. Flowcharts show the whole case management process from beginning to end, as well as some of the common detours it can take along the way. By referring to a flowchart, a supervisor can see what phase the case is in and if the case has taken one of the common detours and needs to get back on track. (An example of a flowchart for vocational rehabilitation can be found in Appendix 3.)

In general, a quality assurance program should focus on "improving the processes for everyone rather than identifying only the problems and unacceptable few. [There should be] continuous improvement rather than static thresholds for quality indicators."[64] Thus, an internal quality control program should not merely focus on identifying unacceptable performance, but it should also be used to improve the overall quality of service delivered to the client and should increase the customer satisfaction of the referral source.

CUSTOMER SATISFACTION SURVEYS

To monitor customer satisfaction, case management providers routinely send out customer satisfaction surveys, often with the final report on a case that is closing. Some of these surveys are also sent to clients. Usually, Likert scale–type questions with five possible rankings from poor to excellent are used.[65] Following are questions that often are asked:

- "Did your case manager return your calls promptly?
- "Was it easy to reach your case manager?
- "Was your case manager knowledgeable about your particular needs?
- "Did you feel your case manager was concerned about you?
- "How would you rate your relationship with your case manager?
- "How would you rate your overall satisfaction with the case management program?"[66]

In implementing a quality assurance program, attention must be paid to all details of the operation because case managers do not work in a vacuum. Their performance is de-

BOX 18-1

KEY ELEMENTS TO INCLUDE ON INTERNAL QUALITY CONTROL CHECKLISTS

- *Opening of cases.* Is approval from the referral source documented? Have screening criteria been properly applied? Is the rationale for opening the case documented?
- *Client consent form.* Is this signed and dated by the client or his or her representative?
- *Timeliness of reports.* Are reports being written at appropriate intervals (e.g., every 30 days)? Are they being typed and mailed soon after they are written or dictated?
- *Adherence to other time frames.* Some firms have very definitive time frames for such things as initial contact with client/family (e.g., within 24 hours of referral), completion of the initial assessment (e.g., within 14 working days of referral), and so on.
- *Compliance with standard report format.* Do all reports follow the standard format required by the company according to the type of report?
- *Accuracy and validity of cost-savings calculations.* Are the correct tabulation and format being used? Do the cost savings appear to be based on valid information? Have short-term and long-term savings been documented separately?
- *Content of reports.* Does information appear to be complete and relevant? Is information repetitious of previous reports? Is each major body system addressed in the initial assessment? For progress reports, have all authorized activities been completed or addressed? Is there written justification if some activities have not taken place?
- *Responsive and reasonable recommendations.* Do the recommendations flow from the body of the report, and are they reasonable in terms of what is happening on the case? Are they reasonable in terms of costs, available alternatives, number of hours for completion, and time frames? Are authorizations of recommendations from the referral source documented?
- *Benefits expectations.* Are reasonable benefits exceptions requested and authorized by the referral source? Are the benefits exceptions justified by the facts on the case? Is the authorization documented in case notes? Are the time frames and duration of benefits exceptions monitored appropriately?
- *Case notes.* Are all billable activities documented in case notes? Do the case notes match the billing? Are the case notes sufficiently descriptive but not overly detailed?
- *Billing.* Is the length of the time billed appropriate for the activity (e.g., client interviews last no longer than 1 to 2 hours, initial reports are written in 2 to 4 hours, progress reports take 1 to 2 hours, correspondence takes 0.50 hour)?
- *Provider placement and negotiation.* Have client needs been adequately matched with a provider that has the resources to address them? Have reasonable rates been negotiated with the provider? Would it be beneficial to explore additional providers before making a recommendation?
- *Monitoring quality of care.* Has a proper placement been coordinated, and is the client being monitored for the appropriateness of the placement? Is the provider complying with commonly accepted standards of care or service? Is the client in a safe setting? Could the client safely be moved to a lower level of care?
- *Case closure.* Has the recommendation for case closure been made in a timely manner? Is the case closure summary brief but descriptive? Are cost savings as a result of case management documented?

pendent on the quality of training, supervision, support staff, office equipment, software, and office systems available through the company. Although only internal quality control for casework is covered in this chapter, systems must be in place for quality assurance of other aspects of the business.

Whether a case manager uses a flowchart or a checklist or frequently screens all case management activity, it is important to remember the importance of internal quality control. This should not merely focus on identifying unacceptable performance but also should be used to improve the overall quality of services. In this way, the client can be assured of assistance in managing health care needs, the payer can be assured that the money spent on case management and in funding further health care for the patient is money well spent, and the case manager will obtain satisfaction from his or her work and take pride in his or her accomplishments as a case manager.

SUGGESTED READINGS

Hodge M: Supervising case managers, *Psychosocial Rehab J* 12(3):51-59, 1989.

Meeks K, Balfour J, Merritt R, Siefker JM: Guidelines for supervision of medical case management, *NARPPS J News* 6(6):251-255, 1991.

References are found at the end of the book.

CHAPTER 19

OUTCOMES MANAGEMENT

EVALUATING CASE MANAGEMENT

The days are long gone when case management firms could merely assert the value of their services without data substantiating these claims. This business is now so competitive that referral sources want specific and defensible information on the value of the case management programs they purchase, especially on how health care outcomes are affected. The information from these evaluations is used, in turn, to improve and maximize the effectiveness of the case management program.

Data on the effectiveness of a case management program are valuable to the case management firm because they help to assess where the firm stands in relation to its competitors. This information can be used quite effectively as a marketing tool. Indeed, it is difficult to be competitive in marketing and making bids on requests for proposals (RFPs) without having this information. Referral sources are definitely in a show-me mode and no longer accept trust-me statements from firms that are trying to market services to them.

It has been observed that "a critical challenge of this area is establishing common, if not universal standards and criteria to measure outcomes."[67] The following discussion focuses on some essential components of an effective evaluation of a case management program.

Early Identification of Clients

Most referral sources and rehabilitation professionals now recognize the value of early identification of cases with potential to benefit from case management.[68] If the case management program does not have effective systems in place for assisting referral sources with early identification of cases, it will not be competitive. Whether cases are identified through utilization review or file reviews at the referral source's office, they need to be evaluated against screening criteria that effectively identify cases with potential to benefit. The screening criteria not only must avoid having cases fall through the cracks but also must guard against overreferral, which is a cost driver by itself. (See Appendix 1 for examples of screening criteria.)

Evaluation of Cost Savings

Not every case will have cost savings, but the aggregate of cases should show a significant cost savings. The cost savings must be accurate, defensible, and based on the reality of the case. These data should be constantly updated by referral source and for the firm as a whole. The data should be broken down by type of case (e.g., organ transplants, high-risk neonates) or by line of insurance, such as workers' compensation or health insurance. A number of software programs are available to sort and develop reports using such data quickly and accurately. However, these systems are only as good as the information they receive. For this reason, particular attention has to be paid to training case managers and supervisors to evaluate cost savings accurately and realistically.

Evaluation of Benefits Exceptions

Evaluating the effectiveness of making benefits exceptions will assist the referral source in making permanent changes to the benefit plan that will result in more appropriate, less costly care. It may also be valuable in assisting the referral source in developing a fee schedule for the new additions to the benefit plan.

Client Satisfaction

Client satisfaction is a key issue in measuring quality and outcomes.[69] To this end, case management companies sometimes send out questionnaires to all clients/families on case closure. This subjective feedback is then tabulated as a measure of client/family satisfaction. Client satisfaction not only improves the public relations (PR) of the referral source but may also improve client responsibility regarding their health care and its costs.

OUTCOMES MEASUREMENT

Referral sources also want to know that health care outcomes are improving as a result of case management and that referrals are being made to providers with a proven track record of quality outcomes. Effecting positive outcomes has a very direct impact on health care costs that often cannot be seen from the calculations of dollar savings on individual cases. Outcomes have an overall impact on the costs of the aggregate of cases.

A number of tools for measurement of outcomes have emerged from the rehabilitation field. These include the Uniform Data System for Medical Rehabilitation's Functional Independence Measure (FIM), Formations in Health Care Inc.'s Level of Rehabilitation Scale (LORS), the Rehabilitation Quality Information (RQI) Network, Short Form-36 Health Survey (SF-36), Rehabilitation Institute of Chicago Functional Assessment Scale (RIC-FAS), and the Functional Assessment Measure (FAM).[70] Although these tools may be highly useful, case managers should not rely too heavily on any one of them because they all have limitations.[71]

Outcomes statistics should be an important component in referral of clients to providers. If a health care agency or facility is not tracking outcomes or will not make outcomes data public, that should be a red flag to the case manager in making a decision to recommend a particular provider. Length of stay, ability to live independently, number of rehospitalizations, morbidity, and ability to return to work should be among the outcomes data available for inspection by the case manager.

If the case manager has a familiarity with outcomes measurement tools, he or she should request information on which tool is being used by the facility. Outcomes measurement tools vary in their effectiveness with some clients and some medical conditions.

Some caution should be used in evaluating a provider's outcomes data. Providers that specialize in chronic patients who are very sick will have less positive outcomes data. When evaluating the data of competing providers, it is necessary to make sure that like programs are being compared and similar data collection and reporting methods are being used.[72] To fairly compare outcomes between providers, risk adjustment methodologies may need to be used. To get the complete story behind the statistics, it is helpful to examine the issues of admission criteria to the program, whether client progress is measured by functional improvements, how client employment is defined, and whether the program follows clients after discharge to ascertain if improvement is sustained.

Outcomes data can also be used by the case manager as the case is being worked to assess progress and to identify what might be impeding progress. This information can help determine if another care or treatment setting would be appropriate and what kind of program modifications can be made within the current health care setting to make it more effective.

In looking at outcomes data for a particular provider, case managers should be sure that the pool of clients on which the facility or agency is reporting is large enough to be statistically significant. Very small numbers may not accurately reflect true outcomes that can be expected. If providers are using different outcomes measurement tools, it may be impossible to compare data effectively.

SUGGESTED READINGS

A brief look at rehab outcomes measures for case managers, *Case Management Advisor* 5(4):49-51, 1994.

Kurowski B: Cancer carve outs and outcomes measurement programs: an emerging paradigm, *Med Interface* 9(11):81-84, 1996.

No yardstick for measuring CM outcomes yet—but change is on the way, *Case Management Advisor* 5(10):133-137, 1994.

Outcomes measurement tools can boost your CM efforts, ensure better patient oversight, *Case Management Advisor* 5(4):46-49, 1994.

Putting outcomes data to work for you: how to show effectiveness of CM intervention, *Case Management Advisor* 5(6):79-80, 1994.

Putting outcomes data to work for you, *Case Management Advisor* 6(6):79-80, 1995.

Romaine DS: Outcomes measurements—tools for case management decisions, *Continuing Care* 14(2): 34-38, 1995.

Understanding outcomes data to make informed CM decisions, *Case Management Advisor* 6(6):77-78, 1995.

References are found at the end of the book.

PART IV
RELATED ASPECTS OF CASE MANAGEMENT

CHAPTER 20
VOCATIONAL REHABILITATION

Case managers are often asked to provide vocational rehabilitation services on workers' compensation cases and sometimes on long-term disability cases. Vocational rehabilitation has many components and theories. This chapter gives only a brief overview of vocational rehabilitation as it pertains to the case manager. (A flowchart of the vocational rehabilitation process is located in Appendix 3.)

In general, the focus of this chapter is workers' compensation work, although much of what is presented may also apply to long-term disability cases. The basic information presented here is very generic. One must keep in mind that vocational rehabilitation varies considerably from state to state and among federal jurisdictions. Before starting any workers' compensation vocational rehabilitation work, the case manager must become thoroughly familiar with the requirements of the state or federal jurisdiction.

REHABILITATION IN WORKERS' COMPENSATION

Rehabilitation in workers' compensation is defined by the Rehabilitation Committee of the Southern Association of Workmen's Compensation Administrators as:

> . . . the cost effective case management by a skilled professional who understands the implications of the medical and vocational services necessary to facilitate an injured worker's expedient return to **suitable gainful employment** with a minimal degree of disability.[73]

From this definition, it is clear that vocational rehabilitation and return-to-work assistance are considered integral aspects of case management.

Vocational rehabilitation on workers' compensation cases is usually aimed at getting the injured worker back to work in some capacity or establishing the employability of an injured worker. Because workers' compensation is an insurance system, the focus is on restoration of loss rather than actualization of the client's vocational potential. For this reason, a hierarchy of return-to-work priorities is usually followed. In developing any return-to-work plan, vocational rehabilitation counselors (VRCs) or case managers must start with the first priority in the hierarchy and must eliminate it and each subsequent one before going on to the next. The following is a generic list of return-to-work priorities, which will vary somewhat according to the workers' compensation system:

- Job at the time of injury with the employer at the time of injury
- Modified version of the job at the time of injury with the employer at the time of injury
- New job based on transferrable skills with the employer at the time of injury

- Job at the time of injury with a new employer
- Modified version of the job at the time of injury with a new employer
- New job based on transferrable skills with a new employer
- New job with a new employer based on skills acquired through on-the-job training (OJT)
- New job with a new employer based on skills acquired through formal training
- Self-employment

When one mentions vocational rehabilitation for injured workers, the first thing that comes to mind tends to be retraining, especially formal schooling. However, these return-to-work priorities indicate that retraining is one of the last options considered.

STEPS IN THE PROCESS

Vocational rehabilitation begins with an initial assessment that focuses on both medical and vocational information. The client is given a complete interview, including a work history, using forms that are similar to those in Appendix 3. (More detailed information on taking a work history is contained in Chapter 21 on vocational evaluation.)

Following the initial interview with the client, the case manager usually visits the employer at the time of injury to discuss return-to-work options and to perform an on-site job analysis (JA). To save time, sometimes the JA and the discussion of return-to-work options take place over the phone. The purpose of this contact is to explore the first three return-to-work priorities and to obtain information about the requirements of the job, especially physical capacities, skills, and working conditions.

The most accurate information for JAs usually is obtained by actually observing the job. However, there may be times when it is impractical to do this, and the case manager must rely on the report of others regarding the job. When obtaining a JA through an interview process rather than observation, the case manager should ask both the client and the supervisor about the job. Performing a JA usually involves completion of a detailed form that describes all pertinent characteristics of the job. (See Appendix 3 for an example of such a form.) Sometimes, jobs are also videotaped or photographed as part of JAs.

A transferrable skills analysis will also be performed to determine what jobs the client might be able to perform based on skills acquired through previous work history and education. (More information on transferrable skills analysis can be found in Chapter 21.) Job analyses are also obtained for any jobs based on transferrable skills that are identified. These can be obtained from files of JAs that most firms providing vocational rehabilitation keep on hand. They may also be obtained by visiting or phoning employers.

Once all relevant JAs have been obtained, the case manager takes them to the attending physician for review and signature. Sometimes, to save time and costs, JAs are faxed or mailed to the physician. In addition to approving or disapproving the job, the attending physician may also suggest possible job modifications that would allow the client to perform the job. Case managers should come armed with ideas for job modifications to discuss with the physician.

If the physician has approved one or more of the JAs, the client is considered employable and may not be eligible for additional services. At this point, the case manager or VRC may write a report that includes an **employability statement** indicating what jobs the client can perform and whether or not these jobs exist within the client's local labor market. To show that a client is employable, it is sometimes necessary to do a **labor market survey (LMS).** This survey consists of calling local employers to ask them if they have had job openings within the last year or anticipate having openings that the client would be able to fill. (A form for performing LMS is located in Appendix 3.)

RETURN TO WORK

Arranging for Job Modifications

If the injured worker is released to return to work at the employer at the time of injury, the case manager or VRC will often facilitate the client's return to work. This will include making arrangements for any job modifications that are needed. Sometimes, clients return to work on a transitional basis, beginning with part-time, light-duty work and gradually working into full duties. Often, the case manager will monitor this **transitional return-to-work** plan until the client returns to work full time. If extensive job modifications are needed, a rehabilitation engineering consultant may be called in to assist. Many job modifications are minor, however, and can be easily arranged.

Referral to Work Hardening

Facilitating the client's return to work may also include a referral to work hardening to physically prepare the client for the physical demands of the job. Clients often become deconditioned during a lengthy recovery period. If they are going to return to a physically demanding job, they may have to undergo conditioning exercises to avoid reinjury. Work hardening programs usually last for a few weeks, during which a simulation of the physical requirements of the job is made to prepare the client for the rigors of the actual job. It is part of a case manager's job to research work hardening programs to select one that best meets the client's needs in the most cost-efficient manner.[74]

Vocational Counseling and Exploration

If the client does not possess any transferrable skills that would enable him or her to be employable, the VRC or case manager often will develop a **vocational rehabilitation plan.** This process begins with vocational counseling and exploration with the client and may involve vocational testing or a **vocational evaluation.** (See Chapter 21 for more detailed information on vocational evaluation.) Vocational evaluation is used to further assess the client's vocational interests, aptitudes, abilities, and temperament to assist him or her in developing appropriate vocational goals.

Vocational counseling and exploration involve meeting with the client to go over vocational rehabilitation options under the workers' compensation system, to present test results, and to discuss vocational options and develop goals. Often, the client is given assignments as part of this process. These may include going to the library to look up information in various reference books or visiting training programs to obtain materials and discuss options. The goal of vocational exploration is to empower the client to make informed choices in selecting job goals and determining the best means for achieving them.

Selecting a Job Goal

In selecting a job goal, close attention must be paid to the return-to-work priorities listed previously. A lower priority cannot be selected unless the previous ones have been eliminated. Once a job goal has been selected, the case manager and client must determine how it is to be achieved. Job placement must be considered before training. Some jobs are entry level and require only very basic skills. Job placement activities are sometimes performed by a job placement specialist who is employed by the vocational rehabilitation firm. (Some jurisdictions do not allow for job placement assistance, so the client is referred to public sector agencies, such as the Employment Service or the Division of Vocational Rehabilitation, for assistance.) Some of the activities that are used to assist a client in finding work include the following:

- Résumé development
- Teaching and coaching to improve job-seeking skills
- Finding job leads and giving them to the client to pursue
- Educating employers on incentives for hiring people with disabilities
- Follow-up with employer and client after job placement to assure job retention

On-the-Job Training. On-the-job training (OJT) must be considered before formal training. An OJT is advantageous because a client is gaining work experience while participating in it. Sometimes, OJTs also result in permanent jobs with the OJT employer. OJTs are sought by contacting employers who are looking for workers. Often, there are financial incentives for employers to train someone on the job rather than hiring an experienced worker. These incentives may include exemption from workers' compensation premiums, not having to pay wages, and tax credits for hiring a worker with a disability.

So that an OJT does not become a way for an employer to have a "cheap pair of hands," a formal OJT agreement usually is written. This indicates the length of the OJT and the learning objectives that are to be achieved at various intervals during the OJT. The OJT agreement is signed by the OJT employer, the client, and the case manager or VRC and becomes a binding contract for all parties.

Formal Retraining. Formal retraining is considered next. A suitable training facility has to be located that offers training for the job goal within the time and monetary constraints of the workers' compensation system. Most workers' compensation systems will not allow more than 1 or 2 years of training and have a cap on the amount of money that can be spent. If the training facility is not well known in the area, the case manager should also check to see if it is accredited and possibly check to see whether local employers will hire its graduates.

WRITING THE FORMAL VOCATIONAL REHABILITATION PLAN

Once the job goal and the means to obtain it have been identified, the case manager must determine whether the job is physically appropriate for the client and exists within the client's local labor market. A JA of the job goal is obtained and sent to the attending physician for review and approval. If the JA is approved, the case manager performs an LMS to see whether jobs related to the goal exist in the labor market.

If a labor market exists, the case manager will then write a formal vocational rehabilitation plan that contains all relevant information required by the referral source so that it can be approved. Many workers' compensation jurisdictions have very specific guidelines regarding the elements that have to be included in a vocational rehabilitation plan for it to be approved. These usually include the following:

- Start and end dates for the plan
- A breakdown of costs that will be associated with the plan
- Rationale for the return-to-work priority chosen and the priorities that were eliminated
- Job goal with *Dictionary of Occupational Titles* (DOT) title, DOT number, and *Guide for Occupational Exploration* (GOE) code
- A complete description of how the job goal is to be obtained
- A JA for the job goal approved by the attending physician
- An LMS
- Brochures or catalogs from the training facility
- A list of responsibilities for the client, VRC, OJT employer, referral source, and others; this list is signed by each of the parties and becomes a binding contract.

Once the vocational rehabilitation plan has been submitted and approved, the case manager will monitor the client's progress and provide assistance in completing it successfully. At the end of the plan, some jurisdictions may allow for job placement activities. If job placement is not a part of the vocational rehabilitation program, the client may be referred to the state employment service, and the case manager will write an employability statement. The employability statement is included in a closing report that documents whether the client is able to work.

SUGGESTED READINGS

Deneen LJ, Hessellund TA: *Vocational rehabilitation of the injured worker,* San Francisco, 1981, Rehab Publications.

Deneen LJ, Hessellund TA, eds: *Counseling the able disabled,* San Francisco, 1986, Rehab Publications.

Deutsch PM, Sawyer HW: *A guide to rehabilitation,* New York, 1990, Matthew Bender.

Get involved early to reduce client's workers' comp costs, speed return to work, *Case Management Advisor* 5(12):161-164, 1994.

Siefker JM, ed: *Vocational evaluation in private sector rehabilitation,* Menomonie, Wisc, 1992, The Rehabilitation Resource.

References are found at the end of the book.

CHAPTER 21
VOCATIONAL EVALUATION

Vocational evaluation is often included as part of a vocational rehabilitation program. **Vocational evaluation** is defined as a process "directed at determining current and potential client functioning for purposes of identifying occupations that could be opened up to the client through the provision of rehabilitation services."[75] This process may include a variety of functions, such as taking a vocational history, transferrable skills analysis, physical capacities evaluation, job tryouts, or work samples, but it is most often associated with vocational testing. All of these components or a combination of one or more may be used in vocational evaluation. The only essential component is taking a vocational history, which normally precedes the other components. At times, it is not necessary to go beyond taking the vocational history.

Basic functions of vocational evaluation are often conducted by rehabilitation counselors or case managers. These individuals will usually take a vocational history, perform transferrable skills analyses, and give some basic tests. Rehabilitation counselors and case managers who are skilled in vocational evaluation may perform the other components as well. Most, however, will prefer to refer clients to special vocational evaluation programs or centers for additional testing, job tryouts, and work samples. Vocational evaluation centers may exist as stand-alone programs or may be in conjunction with other rehabilitation programs, such as sheltered workshops, work adjustment programs, or job training facilities.

Evaluations in these facilities are generally conducted by vocational evaluators. These professionals may come from a variety of backgrounds. They will have a minimum of a bachelors degree and preferably a masters degree in one of several disciplines, including vocational evaluation, rehabilitation counseling, or clinical psychology. In making referrals to vocational evaluators, the case manager should check credentials carefully. Some will also be designated as Certified Vocational Evaluators (CVE) or Certified Rehabilitation Counselors (CRC).

VOCATIONAL HISTORY

To take a vocational history, most VRCs or case managers will use a special form with designated data fields for the information needed. This form often is an extension of the forms that case managers use for the initial interview. The main difference is that the form includes information on work history and educational background. (See Appendix 3 for an example of this type of form.) A complete **work history** will include name of employer, job title, tasks performed, tools and equipment used, years worked, qualifications for the job, and the reason why the job ended.

It is important to obtain information about every job that the individual has held for the last 15 or 20 years. (Jobs that were held farther back than that are usually not considered to be relevant for transferrable skills because most occupations have changed significantly in that amount of time.) Some clients may be aware that they can be deemed employable in occupations that they no longer want to perform and may make a conscious decision to withhold information about particular jobs. Therefore, it is important that the case manager ask the client to account for all periods of unemployment. Not only does this encourage the client to give a complete work history, but also other valuable information, such as periods of incarceration, may be obtained.

Some clients are poor historians, making it necessary to question them carefully to obtain complete information. Sometimes, it is helpful to have the client complete the vocational history sections of the initial interview form at home. That way, the client will have the opportunity to search through personal records to obtain more complete information.

The educational history section is especially significant because the client may have acquired vocational skills that have never actually been used in jobs. If these skills are not too old, they may be considered as transferrable or may be updated with short-term training.

A vocational history may also include a discussion of the client's expressed interests and personal assessment of his or her own skills and abilities. This has to be used with caution, however, because the client's preferences may be irrelevant if he or she is employable in some occupation for which he or she is reasonably qualified by previous experience or training.

In many cases, the vocational history may provide sufficient information about the client to develop a return-to-work plan, and further vocational evaluation components may not be necessary. The vocational history may indicate that the client may return to the job at the time of injury with or without modifications, or it may indicate that the client is qualified for other occupations at the employer at the time of injury.

TRANSFERRABLE SKILLS ANALYSIS

If it does not appear that the client can return to the job at the time of injury or the employer at the time of injury, a transferrable skills analysis may be useful. A transferrable skills analysis is a systematic process for using the vocational history to identify additional jobs that the client can perform based on skills acquired through previous employment.

Using the vocational history, the case manager needs to look up each job in the *Dictionary of Occupational Titles* (DOT)[76] or the *Classification of Jobs* (COJ)[77] or both to make a written profile of each job according to general educational development (GED), aptitudes, specific vocational preparation (SVP), interests, temperament, and physical requirements. (See Appendix 3 for a description of DOT codes and some basic information about the DOT and the COJ.) This profile is then matched to other jobs that require similar characteristics. There are a number of computer job-matching software programs available to assist with this, or the case manager may use the DOT and the COJ. A complete description of how to analyze transferrable skills is beyond the scope of this book, and the reader is referred to *Vocational Assessment: Evaluating Employment Potential*[78] for additional information.

PHYSICAL CAPACITIES EVALUATION

An appropriate job goal cannot be obtained without knowing the physical capacities of the client. This is often accomplished by requesting the attending physician or panel examiners to complete a **physical capacities evaluation (PCE)** form. (See Appendix 3 for an example of this type of form.) Sometimes, it is advantageous to refer the client to a facility that provides performance-based PCEs. Some vocational evaluation programs include this service, but more often, it is provided by a physical therapy facility. Regardless of which type of PCE is used, objective information on physical capacities is an integral part of any vocational evaluation because realistic job goals cannot be developed without it.

VOCATIONAL TESTS

Tests may either be psychometrics (paper and pencil tests) or performance tests. Performance tests use hands-on methods for assessment, but they do not simulate actual jobs. They tend to measure a single trait, such as manual dexterity or keyboarding speed, as opposed to work samples which may evaluate many traits simultaneously.

Standardized testing is are used most often in vocational evaluation. These tests are distinguished from the kind of informal tests that are given in school because they compare the person taking the test to a norm group.[79] A norm group is a population of individuals who were given the test when it was being developed. The populations used for norm groups are usually matched to the general population of the United States so that they comprise a representative sample of the kind of individuals against whom the person being tested will be competing in real life situations, such as school or jobs. The scores from the norm group form a range of scores, or norms. These are generally given as percentiles and sometimes as IQs, academic grade level, or other scores. Using norms, the client can be compared with others to ascertain whether he or she is likely to be able to perform certain jobs successfully or to complete vocational training.[80]

Some of the main types of vocational testing are described in the sections that follow.

Interest Inventories

These are used to assess the similarity of a client's interests to the interests of an occupational grouping. Interest inventories are valuable in career counseling as a starting point in identifying jobs and training goals. These tests, however, do not measure a client's ability to actually perform a job. Some examples of interest inventories are the Career Assessment Inventory and the Wide Range Interest-Opinion Test (WRIOT).

Intelligence Testing (IQ Tests)

IQ tests measure basic learning ability or intelligence, especially as it relates to ability to perform well in school. David Wechsler defines intelligence as "the aggregate or global capacity of the individual to act purposefully, to think rationally, and to deal effectively with the environment."[81]

IQ tests are used when a medical condition, such as a head injury, may have affected learning ability or when new training or education is being considered. In recent decades, IQ tests have come under much fire because scores are considered to be influenced by the dominant culture. Therefore, they should be used with caution with members of minority groups. Some examples of IQ tests are the Wechsler Adult Intelligence Scale-Revised (WAIS-R) and the Revised Beta Examination.

Academic Achievement Tests

Achievement tests measure the client's existing academic functioning. Scores are usually given as grade levels or percentages for reading, spelling, mathematics, and other functions. These tests are used during career counseling when new training or education is being considered or when an occupational goal is being selected. Some examples of achievement tests are the Wide-Range Achievement Test 3 (WRAT-3) and the Peabody Individual Achievement Test-Revised.

Aptitude Tests

These tests measure ability that is believed to indicate a client's capacity for learning a skill or knowledge.[82] They are used during career counseling when new training or education is being considered or when an occupational goal is being selected. A large range of these tests is available to measure a large number of aptitudes. Some examples of aptitude tests are General Aptitude Test Battery (GATB), Differential Aptitude Test Battery (DAT), and Bennett Mechanical Comprehension Test.

Personality Inventories

Personality inventories measure personality traits and temperament factors. They are used to detect psychopathology, to make psychiatric diagnoses, or to assess a client's temperamental match with a particular occupation. These are not always included in vocational evaluations. Their results have been controversial, especially when used with minority groups and for certain purposes. Some examples of personality tests are the Myers-Briggs Type Indicator and the 16 Personality Factors (16PF). Vocational evaluators often do not have the expertise to administer and interpret some of the tests in this category.[83]

WORK SAMPLES

Work samples are hands-on tests involving realistic simulations of jobs.[84] These may be parts of batteries of standardized tests, such as JEVS, TOWER, VALPAR, and McCarron-Dial. Such tests may also be created by the evaluator to address specific needs and may or may not have local norms. Some examples of work samples include taking apart a lock and putting it back together to evaluate spatial perception and mechanical aptitude, and listening to telephone messages on a tape to assess the ability to correctly write down information taken over the phone.

Work samples have the advantage that they appear to be more like real work to the client. Thus, the client may be more accepting of evaluation results using work samples. The major drawbacks to work samples are that they are time consuming to administer and tend to evaluate a number of different aptitudes and skills at the same time, and therefore it is often difficult to know why a client scored poorly on a work sample.

JOB TRYOUTS

Even the best tests, work samples, and PCEs are limited in their ability to simulate the requirements of jobs. At times, the best determination of a person's ability to perform a job or participate in training is a job tryout or job station (also called a situational or community-based assessment). In this situation, a client is given an actual tryout of the job with a real employer. Usually, these tryouts are for a period of time that lasts longer than vocational tests or work samples. Job tryouts may range from a few days to a month or more. By using a job tryout, a case manager can determine if a client has the physical capacities to function indefinitely in a job, if the client has appropriate work behaviors and social skills to be competitively employed, and if the client's job skills are adequate.

Job tryouts are generally used with clients who are severely disabled, such as those with head injuries. Sometimes, they may also be used with clients who are suspected of **malingering** or symptom magnification.

There are agencies or facilities in many cities that specialize in placing clients in job tryouts. Many of these have a group of employers that can provide job tryouts in various occupations. Some of these facilities may be sheltered workshops that provide appropriate job stations inhouse. At times, case managers may have to set up their own job stations by contacting local employers. Because of insurance constraints and wage and hour issues, many employers who are willing to provide job stations are nonprofit. Nonprofit agencies are able to avoid paying wages and workers' compensation premiums on clients on job tryouts because they can group them in the same category as volunteers. To develop a job tryout, it is necessary to have a knowledge of the job or training requirements and performance standards.

Following any combination of interviewing, transferrable skills analysis, testing, work samples, PCEs, and job tryouts, the evaluator or case manager must synthesize all the data collected in order to develop job goals and a return-to-work plan for the client. If the client has been sent to a vocational evaluation unit, the vocational evaluator will synthesize all of this information in a comprehensive report that will list possible job goals and recommendations. The case manager will use this information to empower the client to select appropriate job goals and to develop her or his personal plan for returning to work. This chapter provides a very basic overview of vocational evaluation.

SUGGESTED READINGS

Aiken LR: *Psychological testing and assessment,* Needham Heights, Mass, 1991, Allyn and Bacon.

Alston RJ, Mngadi S: *Vocational aptitude testing in counseling and rehabilitation: historical developments and application issues,* Lexington, Ky, 1990, University of Kentucky.

Siefker JM, ed: *Vocational evaluation in private sector rehabilitation,* Menomonie, Wisc, 1992, The Rehabilitation Resource.

Siefker JM: *Tests and test use in vocational evaluation and assessment,* Menomonie, Wisc, 1996, The Rehabilitation Resource.

Sweetland RC, Keyser DJ, eds: *Tests: a comprehensive reference for assessments in psychology, education and business,* ed 3, Austin, Tex, 1991, Pro-ed.

References are found at the end of the book.

CHAPTER 22

THE AMERICANS WITH DISABILITIES ACT

The Americans with Disabilities Act (ADA) is a piece of federal legislation that was signed into law in 1990. It is a wide-ranging civil rights statute that prohibits discrimination against people with disabilities. It has five titles that address such issues as accessibility and discrimination in public service and public transportation (Title II), public accommodations (Title III), telecommunications (Title IV), and miscellaneous provisions (Title V). These titles relate to some of the services that are used by case managers when working with clients. Title V is significant because one of its provisions is that "insurers may continue to underwrite and classify risks consistent with state laws and entities covered may provide benefits plans based on risk classification."[85]

Case managers, however, are most concerned with Title I, which bars employment discrimination in the public and private sectors and in state and local governments. As of July 26, 1994, all employers with 15 or more employees are required to adhere to its regulations. The ADA is a much more comprehensive piece of legislation than current laws prohibiting discrimination against people with disabilities. It not only prohibits discrimination but requires active measures to provide reasonable accommodation for people with disabilities.

Employers are required to make reasonable accommodations in recruiting, hiring, employing, promoting, and training qualified workers with disabilities. This law applies to all persons with disabilities except for alcoholics and people with drug problems who are still using the substance. Drug tests can still be used to screen out those individuals. Recovering alcoholics and substance abusers who are not current users are covered by the ADA.

The nature of some industries renders them unable to employ many workers with severe physical disabilities. However, they are still required to analyze their jobs for essential job functions and to provide reasonable accommodation whenever possible. Additionally, a large percentage of the people covered by the ADA are not physically disabled (e.g., mentally ill, developmentally disabled, learning disabled, recovering substance abusers). Although many of these individuals have no physical disabilities, they may still have deficits that require accommodation for them to be employable (e.g., poor reading and math skills, poor social skills, unusual behaviors, lack of judgment and reasoning ability).

No longer can employers decree that people with certain disabilities (or any disability) are unable to do certain types of work. Employers must attempt to make reasonable accommodations unless it can be clearly documented that a person cannot perform the "essential functions of a job" or that accommodating a person with a disability would create an undue hardship or would constitute a hazard to people and property. Persons with disabilities have to be considered for employment on an equal basis with other qualified candidates if they can perform the "essential functions of a job."

The ADA is purposefully vague about what constitutes "reasonable accommodations," but case law that has been written since the ADA was written tends to base it on the size and economic status of the company and the cost/benefit ratio of needed accommodations.

ESSENTIAL JOB FUNCTIONS

One of the main provisions of the ADA is that qualified, disabled applicants can only be rejected on the basis of inability to perform "essential job functions." A job function is considered essential if it is the reason that the job exists (e.g., a deaf person could not function as a telephone operator if that job required the ability to hear because hearing people talking on the phone is the main reason the job exists).

Similarly, a function that is not the reason for the job may also be essential if the number of employees performing that function is limited. In this scenario, the employer would not be able to assign the tasks that the person with a disability could not perform to another worker. For example, a machinist position requires the worker to make calibrations of the machine once a week. The calibrations require some overhead reaching that an injured worker cannot perform because of a rotator cuff tear. This function cannot be given to another worker because none of the other workers would have the skills and expertise to perform this function. Thus, even though this function is only performed infrequently, it is an essential one because it cannot be given to another worker.

Functions may also be considered essential because of the amount of time they require. Another type of essential function is one that would have harmful consequences if not performed. A test of whether a function is essential would be if the value of a worker's job would be negated if the function were not performed (e.g., a dyslexic might not be able to be a proofreader because she would experience difficulty in reading and could not perceive errors in text).

In determining essential functions of a job, there is a distinction between being able to perform a task and being able to produce what the job requires. For example, a worker might be unable to lift 50-pound items to a bench to put them in place for work tasks that would be within his capabilities. Although he could not do the lifting task, he could use a lifting device to perform this function. If the purchase of the lifting device was not an undue hardship to the company, it would be considered a reasonable accommodation for the employer to make.

Modern technology is developing more and more assistive devices that are more ergonomically sound and enable workers with disabilities to perform functions that were previously beyond their physical capacities. If the worker can produce the end result that is required even though the method is different, he or she is considered able to perform an essential function.

THE ADA'S IMPLICATIONS FOR CASE MANAGERS

The ADA has many implications for the case manager who is handling workers' compensation cases. Mainly, it has been used quite effectively by injured workers to force their employers to make reasonable accommodations to return them to work. Since returning an injured worker to the job and the employer at the time of injury is the most cost-efficient strategy, the ADA has made the job of the case manager easier in many respects. Because of this, "the rehabilitation case manager may now serve as an injured worker's advocate, without necessarily posing the threat of being a disservice to the employer or its [workers' compensation] carrier."[86]

Job Modifications

Most employers who are covered by the ADA are aware of its implications and are willing to explore the possibility of job modifications. The case manager who is working with injured workers needs to be able to effectively analyze jobs (see Chapter 20 for more information) to determine their essential functions and possible reasonable accommodations that could be made. He or she also needs to be creative with respect to identifying possible ways that jobs can be modified.

It should be noted that many accommodations cost very little or nothing. Often, they involve such simple things as rearranging workstations or reallocating the duties of several workers to eliminate the ones that the person with a disability cannot perform and to give him or her additional duties to fill in the gap left by the duties that were eliminated. Some accommodations make the workplace more safe and ergonomically sound for all the workers, thus reducing workers' compensation claims.

Job modifications can involve special tools that are designed to reduce vibration or movements that aggravate the disabling condition. They can be simple apparatuses such as a stool placed in front of a worker to be a footrest to take some of the pressure off her back while she is standing. At the opposite extreme, job modifications can include installing elevators, ramps, special computers, and other costly items. Because it is often difficult to determine how jobs can be modified, the case manager may wish to call in one of the numerous ADA consultants who specialize in job analysis and job modifications. This type of consultant may also have useful information about public funding sources (some workers' compensation systems, the state Division of Vocational Rehabilitation) available to assist with job modifications.

A frequent objection to making an accommodation is that it would constitute an undue hardship. This issue needs to be carefully negotiated with the employer. Very large employers who are well capitalized would find it difficult to claim undue hardship under most circumstances, but this becomes problematic when the employer is small and is not doing well financially. If alternate funding for the job modification can be obtained, this objection can usually be overcome.

Safety Issues

Safety issues also deserve careful consideration. There is a difference between safety concerns that might pose a one in a million risk of injury and ones that pose a clear and present danger. Employers sometimes raise safety issues when their real reason for concern lies in another realm entirely (e.g., they do not want to take back someone who has been a behavior problem at work). It has been noted that "risk must be defined using objective, factual evidence—not subjective perceptions, irrational fears, patronizing attitudes or stereotypes about the nature or effect of a particular disability or of disability generally."[87]

Unions

One concern that employers often have is whether the ADA covers unions. It is true that collective bargaining agreements usually contain very specific provisions about job descriptions and the qualifications of those who hold them. However, unions are now included under the ADA and must also make reasonable accommodations. One concern of unions is that restructuring of jobs to accommodate workers with disabilities will result in nondisabled workers having to do more work that is dangerous, physically taxing, and unpleasant. This type of concern will have to be dealt with in a creative manner. In some cases, assistive devices and ergonomically sound equipment can be introduced to improve the working conditions of all workers.

Implications for Hiring

In helping clients to find new jobs, the case manager also needs to be cognizant of the implications of the ADA for hiring. Employers are required to make their interview process and preemployment screening nondiscriminatory. They must focus on identifying those who are able to perform the essential functions of the job and must not inadvertently eliminate applicants with certain types of disabilities. Employers sometimes base their hiring decisions on test results. Applicants who could otherwise perform a job may be eliminated because they cannot do a test (e.g., an applicant with a back injury might not be able to do a lifting test but would be able to perform the job with the help of a lifting device). Employers must be willing to eliminate or modify tests so that they do not discriminate against workers who are otherwise qualified.

Likewise, employers must make sure that preemployment physicals are based on essential job functions and that nonmedical staff are not making medical judgments on the applicant's ability to perform the job. For example, a vision test could be given only if a certain level of visual acuity were required by the job. When a client is applying for jobs, the case manager should educate him or her on the ADA and may wish to address these issues with employers.

If a case manager is to be involved in vocational rehabilitation, he or she needs to be well acquainted with the ADA and recent case law to be able to educate employers and clients on the ADA and discuss its implications with them. In recent years, there have been a number of excellent training programs and books on the ADA.

SUGGESTED READINGS

Bureau of National Affairs: OSHA draft ergonomic protection standard summary of key provisions, *Occup Safety Health Reporter* 345-348, July 13, 1994.

Frederick LJ: Cumulative trauma disorders—an overview, *AAOHN J* 40(3):113-116, 1992.

Hales T, Bertsche P: Management of upper extremity cumulative trauma disorders, *AAOHN J* 40(3):118-128, 1992.

Lotito MJ, Soltis MJ, Pimentel R: *The Americans with Disabilities Act: a comprehensive guide to Title I,* Northridge, Calif, 1992, Milt Wright & Associates, Inc.

Occupational Safety and Health Administration: *Job hazard analysis,* Washington, DC, 1992, US Government Printing Office.

Pimentel R, Bissonnette D, Lotito MJ: *What managers & supervisors need to know about the ADA,* Northridge, Calif, 1992, Milt Wright & Associates, Inc.

Powers K, Arnstein C: Getting them back to work safely, *Occup Health Safety,* 42-45, 68, Feb 1995.

Rodgers B: *Occupational health nursing concepts and practice,* Philadelphia, 1994, WB Saunders.

Walker JM: The Americans with Disabilities Act and the rehabilitation CM, *Case Manager* 3(3):41-42, 44, 46, 1992.

References are found at the end of the book.

CHAPTER 23

CLIENT PLACEMENT AND PROVIDER NEGOTIATIONS

An important part of cost containment in case management is placing the client in an appropriate care facility and negotiating favorable rates and fees with the provider. Some case managers have personalities that make it easier for them to do the negotiations required; others have to learn basic negotiation skills.

CLIENT PLACEMENT

The first step in client placement is identification of appropriate facilities. This can be accomplished by completing the Patient Care Assessment Form and the Health Care Facility/Agency Questionnaire that are shown in Appendix 2 and can be adapted to meet local needs. These forms are used in conjunction with one another to match a client's health care needs to appropriate health care facilities or agencies that can address them. The Patient Care Assessment Form is completed first to identify the health care needs of the client. It may be completed through interviewing the client/family and with the attending physician and other health care providers.

The goal in using this form is to develop a complete picture of what the client needs in terms of level of care, number of hours recommended, and length of time client is projected to need care. It also addresses types of care required, such as activities of daily living, supervision, medications, pain management, therapies or treatments, and other nursing care. This form also identifies client characteristics in terms of impaired function, behavioral disorders, ability to comply with the treatment program, and family/social support. It addresses issues related to the coverage or noncoverage of some types of care, treatment, supplies, or durable medical equipment (DME).

After completing the Patient Care Assessment Form, the case manager looks for appropriate facilities or agencies that can provide the care that is needed. This is done partially by researching brochures and other information kept on file at the office on various health care agencies and facilities located within the geographic area being served. When the case manager finds a facility or agency that may be appropriate, he or she contacts it to obtain more information. At this point the case manager may complete the Health Care Facility/Agency Questionnaire to ensure that the facility is able to adequately address all issues pertinent to the health and safety of the client. This questionnaire requests information on current licensure, specialty certification, targeted patient population, staffing level, patient/staff ratio, services provided, preferred patient characteristics (e.g., age, diagnosis), costs, and ability to interface with the case manager.

BOX 23-1

METHODS TO ASSESS ANCILLARY SERVICE PROVIDERS

- *Client/family satisfaction.* Ask potential providers if they have references from former clients or families who can be contacted to discuss satisfaction. Facilities may also have results of formal surveys that they can share.
- *Outcomes/effectiveness data.* Ask for statistics on mortality, morbidity, return to work, health restoration, and treatment/care plan goals achieved. Accredited facilities should keep these data and make them available to those who request them. Does this facility produce outcomes that are in line with others that provide similar services? Poor outcome statistics are a red flag that your client may not receive maximum benefit from treatment or care.
- *Infrastructure.* Determine what types of **accreditation** the provider has (e.g., JCAHO, CHAP, and CARF). Ask about the qualifications of the staff and the staff/patient ratio. What is the staff turnover rate? Program stability may be reflected by stable staffing patterns. Who is the medical director? What facilities and services are available? Is there an internal quality control program? Ask to see their risk management protocols.
- *Process.* After making contact with a facility, subjectively evaluate whether they were responsive to your requests and were able to communicate effectively. As a case manager, will you be able to function as part of an interdisciplinary team while your client is a patient? Will you be able to contact individual team members as necessary?
- *Data.* Does the facility report data by both individual and aggregate cases?
- *Compliance with standards.* Does the facility use disease state management, critical pathways, criteria, or quality screens when determining care and treatment protocols? What about variation analysis and interpretation and physician order compliance?

If the health care facility or agency is able to address all the needs of the client in an appropriate manner, the case manager may consider placing the client in its care. When there is a variety of appropriate facilities or agencies in a given geographic area, the case manager may use the Health Care Facility/Agency Questionnaire to comparison shop for prices and negotiate a better rate.

Matching the client's needs to the facility is not the only component in identifying an appropriate placement. To ensure that dollars are used wisely, the case manager may wish to assess the quality of the facility to ensure that the client receives services that are likely to result in recovery or other favorable outcomes. Because facilities vary in the quality of their services, the one with the lowest prices may not be the most cost-efficient option. Box 23-1 describes some ways of assessing quality components and outcome statistics of ancillary service providers.

PROVIDER NEGOTIATIONS

An important component of case management interventions is securing adequate cost savings from provider negotiations. Payers frequently have expectations that case management interventions will secure hard dollar cost savings. These cost savings can be achieved in a variety of ways, including negotiations with providers as well as facilitating appropriate cost-effective client placement.

Negotiation skills should be a component of case management orientation because most new case managers do not come to case management with experience in negotiation. Effective negotiation occurs most often when it is incorporated as a key component of the case management process. To be an effective negotiator, the case manager must have a good working knowledge of the goals, medical/psychosocial background, and expectations of the payer, client, and health care providers. Additionally, the case manager must be familiar with alternative providers in the area. The case manager who can approach the negotiation process equipped with adequate information on the patient's needs and the health care environment in the area is better able to negotiate fees.

Negotiation with health care providers is most effective when it is approached from a perspective of open, honest communication. The provider frequently has additional information and resources on the equipment or services that are being negotiated. The case manager's goal is not only to obtain cost savings but also to ensure that the client is receiving the most appropriate equipment or service. Collaborative working relationships with providers are essential for long-term case management success.

Each case manager will develop his or her own individual negotiation style. Important negotiation components to remember are to speak in a clear, precise way and outline expectations in an assertive manner.

There are several different types of provider negotiations that may occur within the case management process. These include fee-for-service arrangements, per diem arrangements, case rate negotiations, and rent vs. purchase negotiations.

Fee-for-Service

Most home health care and DME are billed under a fee-for-service arrangement. Case managers frequently will negotiate a flat discount off the cost of the service (e.g., a 15% discount off the list price of a Registered Nurse home visit). It is imperative in these cases to be familiar with what the community norm list price is for any fee-for-service equipment or service.

Case managers can also negotiate flat discounts off procedures or hospital admissions. Some providers will negotiate a flat discount off the total bill for a service in return for prompt (30 day) payments. This is especially beneficial for those providers who do not have a preferred provider network identified.

Per Diem Arrangements

Infusion therapy and hospice care frequently are negotiated under a per diem arrangement. When negotiating infusion therapy pricing for a client, the case manager attempts to secure a discounted price off the list per diem or daily rate for the infusion therapy. Infusion therapy is frequently billed at a per diem rate plus the average wholesale price (AWP) of the drug to be infused. Case managers can frequently negotiate substantial cost savings on infusion therapy from the provider's list price. The per diem rate for the therapy typically includes all supplies, the infusion pump, and the nursing care, although this is usually open to negotiation.

Hospice services are also moving toward a standardized per diem arrangement. The majority of hospice agencies get most of their referrals from the Medicare population. Medicare has a hospice per diem benefit, and most hospice agencies are moving toward standardizing all their clients under this type of arrangement. Hospice per diem arrangements typically include intermittent skilled nursing visits, social worker visits, and home health aide visits, as well as all routine DME, oxygen, and all medications related to the terminal diagnosis. Case managers can negotiate not only on the daily charge but also on the services provided under the per diem arrangement (e.g., asking that 10 hours of respite care a week or a certain number of palliative radiation treatments be included in the hospice package).

Frequently, a per diem rate is a more cost-effective payment structure because of the acuity of services that the home-based terminal patient requires. The case manager must be very familiar with the client's status and the disease process before using this type of payment structure. Under a per diem structure, a daily charge is billed regardless of what services are provided. If a patient has multiple needs and will require many services in the home, a per diem structure is more cost effective, but if the patient will not require multiple services, this structure is not cost effective.

Case Rate Negotiations

These negotiations are frequently performed for major procedures (e.g., organ transplants or bone marrow transplants). The case manager works with the facility or program to develop an all-inclusive case rate for the procedure. The case manager must be familiar with the procedure before entering into the negotiation process and have a clear idea of what the case rate should include. Typical case rate negotiations for an organ transplant may include such items as organ acquisition, transplantation, acute inpatient admission, and 6 weeks of outpatient follow-up.

Purchase Versus Rental Negotiations

Most DME and oxygen supplies can be rented or purchased from the provider. The case manager, again, must be very familiar with the client's situation to determine the cost savings from purchasing versus renting equipment. Most major DME items, such as electric wheelchairs, can be purchased with a flat fee-for-service, negotiated discount. For the patient who may require an item of DME for an indeterminate amount of time, monthly rental may be more appropriate. Case management can negotiate discounts off the monthly rental price and can also request that the monthly rental be applied toward the purchase price of a particular piece of DME.

ADDITIONAL CONSIDERATIONS

Sometimes, there will be only one appropriate facility or supplier, but it is helpful in negotiations if there is more than one place from which to choose. Some facilities or suppliers will not be undersold by their competitors. Negotiating a favorable rate will depend on a number of factors:

- *Referral source's experience with provider.* If the referral source has been a frequent purchaser of services from the facility, it is often possible to negotiate volume discounts. Similarly, if the case management firm or case manager refers a lot of cases to the provider, he or she may be able to use that as leverage to obtain discounts.
- *Amount of competition.* If a provider has a great deal of competition and facilities tend to be underused, there may be some incentive to lower prices. The case manager can mention that competitors are charging less or that as everyone charges the same, the client will likely choose a more conveniently located competitor if a more favorable rate cannot be negotiated.
- *Ask for additional services.* If the vendor is not willing to reduce prices, the case manager can ask to have additional services included.

Whenever possible, the case manager should have more than one facility or provider to compare prices and services. Because providers vary considerably in price, quality, and services, it is helpful to chart out or list what each provider has to offer so that an objective comparison can be made.

Although the goal is to obtain the best care or treatment for the least amount of money, the client/family should not be left out of the equation. The case manager must always keep in mind the empowerment of the client. The client's and family's needs and wishes should be considered in any placement. These may include convenience of geographic location and social and esthetic issues. The attending physician may also have preferences regarding health care facilities and agencies, so he or she should be consulted as well. Balancing these factors may be complex.

SUGGESTED READINGS

Schaffer CL: Case management law: shopping for the best price, *Continuing Care* 12(3):34, 1993.

Tips for making the right subacute placement choice, *Case Management Advisor* 5(3):32-34, 1994.

CHAPTER 24
ETHICS IN CASE MANAGEMENT

Ethics in case management is somewhat different from ethics in nursing or social work. Beginning case managers may feel that they are well versed in ethics from their experiences as nurses or social workers, only to find that there are a number of new issues that pertain to case management but not nursing or social work in general. It has been noted, however, that "ethics is inherently intertwined with morality. In the practice of the healthcare professions, ethics traditionally has dealt with the interpersonal level between provider (e.g., case manager) and client, rather than the policy level which emphasizes the good of society. Ethics deals with ferreting out what is appropriate in situations which are labeled 'dilemmas' because there are no really good alternatives and/or where none of the alternatives is particularly desirable. Thus, ethics addresses the judgment of right and wrong or good and bad."[88]

STANDARDS OF PRACTICE

The foundation for any discussion of ethics in case management begins with the standards of practice developed by some organizations to which many case managers belong. Two of those organizations are Case Management Society of America (CMSA) and National Association of Rehabilitation Professionals in the Private Sector (NARPPS).[89,90] These standards of practice cover a broad range of areas, including definitions of case management, goals and philosophy of case management, the role or function of the case manager, the settings in which case management takes place, standards of care, the relationship of the case manager to the client, standards of performance, and other issues. When faced with any ethical dilemmas, the case manager would do well to consult one of these performance standards for guidance.

NARPPS' performance criteria for case managers do not specifically address the subject of ethics but imply that case managers will adhere to the rights of the client and will act as a client advocate by assisting the client in making informed decisions. This will be accomplished by seeking appropriate resources and consultation. In other words, case managers are expected to act in ways that are not contrary to the interests of the client or patient.[91] Also, it is often difficult to determine who the client is when doing case management.[92]

According to CMSA,[93] "case management is guided by the principles of autonomy, beneficence, nonmaleficence, justice and veracity." The case manager must have a commitment to preserving the autonomy, dignity, and privacy of the client by empowering him or her to be a self-advocate who acts appropriately on his or her own behalf or, according to performance criteria, is a component in providing ethical service. CMSA's performance standards contain a basic list of ethical standards that should guide the case manager's practice.[94]

These standards convey that the case manager must respect the dignity, autonomy, and confidentiality of the patient/client. In doing this, the case manager works for the good of the client and seeks to avoid doing harm to the client. A component of this is working to ensure justice for the client or that the client receives what is right and fair. Veracity or ensuring that the truth is told and that the client is adequately informed is a major component in both justice and maintaining a trusting relationship with the client. All of these aspects of ethical case management are critical to the goals of case management and positive outcomes.

CLIENT ADVOCACY

One of the most difficult areas for a case manager often revolves around the issue of client advocacy. Sometimes, it is easy to lose sight of who the client is because the client probably has not requested and is not paying for case management services. When the referral source is paying for the services, it is tempting to always act on their behalf because, on the surface at least, that will please them and result in more referrals.

However, this is a short-sighted point of view. For one thing, the referral source is contracting for case management because it does not have the medical expertise to manage some types of cases. It is not looking for someone to rubber stamp its decisions and do whatever it asks. Referral sources genuinely want additional information that will help them make informed decisions. Insurance companies, especially, are concerned about bad faith claims, in which the claimant or subscriber does not get everything that is medically needed or that he or she is entitled to under the insurance policy. Bad faith claims are costly to the insurance company because of litigation and penalties or punitive damages. They may also create a major public relations problem for the insurance company. Therefore, insurance companies want information from case managers that will help them avoid bad faith claims.

On the other hand, insurance fraud is a common enough occurrence that is very costly to the insurance system and society as a whole. Although it is not the role of the case manager to prevent insurance fraud, the case manager may often be privy to information that indicates that fraudulent or at least wasteful practices are going on. Whether or not to share this information with the referral source is often a difficult dilemma, especially if the consequences of doing so would have seriously detrimental effects on the client or would jeopardize the relationship with the client, thus making the provision of further case management services difficult or impossible.

At times, it is tempting to do what would benefit the referral source more than the client because the referral source is paying for the case management. However, for the sake of everyone concerned, it is important for the case manager to be as neutral, objective, and ethical as possible. Colluding with the referral source to save money by engaging in questionable practices or sacrificing the client's interests in favor of the referral source's interests may please the referral source and result in more business in the short run. However, because of the checks and balances within most systems, case management firms that do this eventually lose out.[95] Claims decisions based on faulty information resulting from inadequate case management services can be successfully appealed and overturned, resulting in increased costs and bad public relations for the referral source.

Regardless of who has contracted for their services, case managers must always remember that the patient and not the referral source is the client. The system works best if the client's needs are addressed in relation to what is covered by the referral source. If the client has needs that are not covered by the referral source, the case manager must research whether they are truly medically necessary and seek other resources to address them. Sometimes, the client may have needs that are not in the medical or vocational realm but are essential for quality of life and medical recovery, nevertheless. Other resources can be sought in the community through churches and nonprofit organizations.

FINANCIAL CONSIDERATIONS

Balancing client needs with the provisions of the benefit plan is often a difficult juggling act. A situation that arises frequently occurs when there is only limited funding for certain needs, such as mental health. If the need is great and the funding is limited, the issue to be addressed is how to get the most for the dollars available. This is where careful research of treatment alternatives and treatment facilities comes in. Good price negotiation skills are also a factor. In this type of scenario, the case manager is often tempted to go with the lowest priced services, yet it is usually true that you get what you pay for, meaning that low priced services or goods may not be adequate to address the client's needs. The case manager must evaluate quality as well as price in making recommendations for treatment facilities, services, and equipment. Doing this is not as simple as it sounds because there are usually many tradeoffs to consider and factors to balance in informed decision making.

Cost shifting is a current trend in medical cost containment. Even though there are other resources who might fund client needs, is it ethical to shift the costs? If a referral source has a fiduciary obligation to fund certain client needs, it may be unethical to shift the costs even if it is possible to do so, thereby increasing the dollar savings that accrue as a result of case management.

Another financial issue is whether to use case manager time and associated costs to look for community resources to address client needs rather than merely leaving it up to the client to fund these needs out-of-pocket or go without. Controlling the costs of case management is a major factor in selling referral sources on the value of case management, yet there is an obligation to assist the client that may go beyond advocacy issues. If the client does not have certain needs met, the medical condition may eventually exacerbate, resulting in more costs to the referral source in the long run.

This brings up the subject of exceptions to medical benefits. Sometimes, requesting exceptions to benefits will clearly result in cost savings (e.g., reducing inpatient days through provision of home health care). At other times, the potential for cost savings may not be so clear (e.g., use of experimental treatments or procedures). Recommending exceptions to benefits has to be done cautiously because there is always a potential for unintended consequences that negate any potential cost savings and may even be cost drivers.

When considering experimental treatments or procedures, the case manager must always weigh the potential harm that could result. The necessity for careful and thorough research of options in case management is a very significant factor in providing ethical services. Accurate and complete information must always be available to make informed choices. The case manager's personal biases regarding certain procedures, treatment modalities, and providers must not unduly influence the information that is obtained and shared with the client.

CONFIDENTIALITY

A frequent subject of concern for case managers is confidentiality. Despite more and more legislation governing privacy, it is often not clear who has a right to certain information. Traditionally, clients have had a right to confidentiality between them and their medical providers or counselors. With the advent of third-party payment systems, clients have had to give up some rights in this regard. It has been noted that "the key in dealing with these ethical questions consists in sorting out the moral duties and obligations that define the moral relationships among the insurers, the professionals and the insureds."[96] In some situations, case managers even have an obligation to violate the client's privacy and report certain things. Workers' compensation systems often have regulations against colluding with the client. This extends to an obligation to report suspected instances of insurance fraud. If the client says, "I will tell you something, but you must promise not to tell the insurance company," the case manager should consider whether confidentiality rights in this case can really be respected. Although there may be compelling reasons for respecting the privacy rights of the client, to do so in some legal jurisdictions may result in the case manager being named in a lawsuit.[97]

At the beginning of the case as part of the initial interview, the case manager should thoroughly explain his or her role, especially regarding confidentiality. In some systems, particularly workers' compensation, the case manager is under an obligation to report all relevant information to the referral source. This type of information will include such things as working and collecting benefits at the same time, but it may not extend to things that have nothing to do with the fiduciary obligations of the workers' compensation system (e.g., a recent abortion).

The client has a right to privacy in regard to matters that are outside the jurisdiction of the referral source. However, distinctions in this area are often unclear. For example, the client may have told a case manager that her children were taken away from her because she is an alcoholic. The client may still appear to be drinking heavily, which is interfering with medical progress or return to work. Even though the alcoholism is unrelated to the industrial injury, it may be hindering the goal of workers' compensation, which is to return the client to work. Obviously, informing the client about confidentiality rights and getting him or her to sign an appropriate release of information form are essential functions in providing ethical case management.

Case managers may also encounter unrelated issues in the course of their work that obligate them to make certain types of reports. For example, although a case manager may not be working with a client's children, he or she may observe conditions that lead to a suspicion of abuse or neglect. In most jurisdictions, professionals are obligated to make reports to the proper authorities when they suspect abuse or neglect.

Another confidentiality issue relates to the use of fax machines and mail. Because written material received through these sources is often handled by nonprofessionals, it is necessary "to take some sort of reasonable precaution . . . to ensure the patient's confidentiality."[98] This may involve such simple actions as writing "confidential" in large letters at the top of the written material.

CLIENT RIGHTS

The client must always be treated as an individual and accorded appropriate rights and respect. This includes respecting the client's cultural, ethnic, or religious heritage. (This is discussed more thoroughly in Chapter 26.) It also involves ensuring that the client has complete information to make informed choices. A critical component of this is educating the client in terms that can be easily understood by him or her. Even though the case manager and the medical providers believe that a certain course of action is the right choice, the client must be allowed the autonomy to make the decision. If the client chooses to make a decision that is unsafe, the case manager should continue to educate the client,[99] but ultimately the client must make the final decision. Families need to be brought into the decision-making process when they will be involved in care or in cases where the patient is not alert and oriented.

Patient choice of treatment facilities and providers also poses an ethical dilemma in case management. When the goal is to save dollars, the client may be transferred to a facility where he or she does not want to be. The facility may not be in a good location, may have a bad reputation in the client's eyes, or may force the client to mingle with people that he or she wishes to avoid. In this scenario, the goal of saving dollars comes into direct conflict with the goal of client empowerment and autonomy. The case manager might resolve this by pointing out to the client the advantages of saving dollars when benefits are limited and coverage may not be available for all services that are needed.

QUALITY OF CARE ISSUES

Other quality of care and collusion issues loom. What should a case manager do when clients are being overmedicated or overtreated? Sometimes, it is the client who is lying to medical providers to obtain drugs or unnecessary treatment. What about physicians who refer their patients to treatment facilities in which they have a financial interest? A case manager would have an ethical responsibility to report situations of this nature.

Conflicts often arise when decisions are made regarding the medical necessity of proposed services and equipment. Often, it is not clear that certain tests and procedures are necessary. In the past, medical costs have been driven to a large extent by physicians' desire to avoid litigation by leaving no stone unturned. This still goes on, but there is danger of the pendulum swinging the other way, causing decision making in favor of cost savings that may be detrimental to the client. In real life, medical necessity is often not easy to determine.

When conflicts arise over medical necessity issues, matters are often settled through appeals processes. The case manager may assist clients and their attending physicians regarding the appeals process whenever a denial is made.

OTHER ETHICAL CONSIDERATIONS FOR CASE MANAGERS

Vendors of other medical goods and services have recognized the influence that case managers have over medical consumption and the associated purchasing power. As a result, case managers have become the targets of widespread marketing efforts by companies selling all sorts of medical products. Case managers need to be cognizant of the ethical implications of accepting finder's fees and other gratuities from vendors or even being the recipient of excessive wining and dining. Being associated with practices of this nature not only is unethical, but it also compromises the basis of case management—that of being an objective professional whose role is to ensure that medical dollars are spent in the most cost-efficient manner.

Right-to-die issues have been prominent in the media for some time, and they are starting to touch the role of the case manager when working with clients who are terminally ill. Sometimes, the wishes of the family, the client, and the medical system are in conflict.[100] The problem is compounded when the client is currently unable to express his or her own wishes on this subject but has discussed this with the case manager in the past. Even if a living will has been written, the family will sometimes choose to ignore it. Should the case manager intervene in this type of situation? There are no easy and clear answers to some of these questions. Each case manager must sort through these situations and act accordingly to her or his own conscience.

Vocational rehabilitation also brings with it a number of ethical dilemmas. A client might want to return to work before he or she is physically able because of extreme financial need. Perhaps he or she is not receiving enough on disability payments to make the mortgage payment and provide for basic family needs. If the client does not return to work, he or she will likely lose his house. The case manager would have to balance this concern with the fact that the client has not made a sufficient recovery to return to work and would be in danger of an exacerbation that might cause him to be permanently disabled from his usual line of work. At the opposite extreme is the employer who wants to use the workers' compensation system to terminate an undesirable employee even though the employer is covered by the ADA and could make reasonable accommodations to return the injured worker to work.

Case managers must always work within applicable laws and regulations and must not collude with anyone to circumvent them. They must always weigh the risks and benefits of following a certain course of action. In the real world, the best course of action is not always clear.

Likewise, the client has the right to take risks both in choosing treatment and facilities and in leisure time activities.[101] This means that the process of empowering the client also includes allowing the client to make mistakes or to do things that are against medical advice. Thus, a major aspect of ethics involves treating the client as an independent entity who has the right to make choices even if they are greatly counter to the opinions of the case manager and the medical establishment. Yet, this philosophy may be in direct conflict with one of the roles of case management, which is cost containment, if the client's decision is likely to become a cost driver.[102]

The number of ethical scenarios that can arise in the course of case management is infinite. Ethical issues are coming more and more to the forefront as new methods for managed care are developed and medical science advances. New technology always brings with it ethical considerations that were not significant previously. A special concern is new or experimental treatments that have not been proven to be effective but are costly. Costly procedures tend to bring up the specter of rationing of care, which is distasteful to many Americans. Ascertaining which clients are likely to benefit from costly procedures is often difficult. Case managers need to do careful research and to coordinate the opinions of medical providers. Ultimately, decisions lie with physicians, referral sources, and clients. The case manager's role is to facilitate communication and information sharing so that informed decisions are made on the part of all parties.

Because ethical dilemmas are notoriously unclear and difficult to analyze, case managers should seek advice from supervisors or colleagues. Bouncing ideas off another person is often an excellent way to become clear about the issues at hand. The best thing a case manager can do, however, is to question his or her own motives. It has been suggested to ask, "Are we really in there for the consumer or is it secondary gain? The real job of today and tomorrow's case managers is educating everyone involved—the treatment team, patient, and consumer—on the best medical decision."[103]

SUGGESTED READINGS

Aguilar FJ: *Managing corporate ethics,* Cary, NC, 1994, Oxford University Press.

Banja JD: Ethics: conflicts of interest (Part I), *Case Manager* 2(4):24, 26, 1991.

Banja JD: Ethics: conflicts of interest (Part II), *Case Manager* 3(1):20, 22, 1991.

Beauchamp T, Childress J: *Principles of biomedical ethics,* ed 4, New York, 1995, Oxford University Press.

Case Management Society of America: CMSA statement regarding ethical case management practice, *J Care Management* 2(2):8-9, 1996.

Frankena WK: *Ethics,* ed 2, Englewood Cliffs, NJ, 1973, Prentice-Hall.

Frommer M: *Ethical issues in health care,* St Louis, 1981, Mosby.

Hudson T: Administrative ethics in the 1990s: CEOs confront payment, access dilemmas, *Hospitals* 66(1):20, 1992.

Kahn KL and others: Comparing outcomes of care before and after implementation of the DRG-based prospective payment system, *JAMA* 264(15):1984-1988, 1990.

McClinton DH: Balancing the issue of ethics in case management, *Continuing Care* 14(5):13-16, 1995.

Reich P: Capitation and ethics, *Med Interface* 9(9):16, 1996.

Saulo M, Wagener RJ: How good case managers make tough choices: ethics and mediation, Part 1, *J Care Management* 2(1):8-15, 51-55, 1996.

Saulo M, Wagener RJ: How good case managers make tough choices: ethics and mediation, Part 2, *J Care Management* 2(2):10-16, 35, 37-38, 1996.

Smith DS: CMSA statement regarding ethical case management practice, *J Care Management* 2(2):8-9, 1996.

Tarvydas V, Maki DR: News from CCMC: ethics for supervisors, *J Care Management* 2(4):42, 1996.

Veatch RM: Allocating health resources ethically: new roles for administrators and clinicians, *Frontiers of Health Services Management* (8)1:3-29, 1991.

References are found at the end of the book.

CHAPTER 25

Disease Management

If case management is the evolutionary step beyond utilization management, disease management may be thought of as the next step beyond case management. However, disease management is still a newly emerging approach in health care, as there are many definitions and models of disease management. The early model of disease management was an outgrowth of pharmaceutical benefit management, but that only involved a defined pharmaceutical regimen for a specific condition and not the entire spectrum of care. Disease management has become a broader, more comprehensive program involving care delivered across multiple settings through an integrated network of providers and other strategic partners to treat a given disease or condition through a planned clinical pathway.

DISEASE MANAGEMENT DEFINED

The essence of case management is disease management, which "refers to patient care across the continuum from well but 'at risk,' to acute episode, through rehabilitation, and back to well but at risk."[104] Disease management "involves a defined condition; it provides a continuum of education to change patient behavior, and it coordinates physician, hospital and home care."[105] Ward and Rieve define it "as the integration of services across the continuum of care to treat a given disease with the goals of improved outcomes and reduced costs. [They go on to say that] A managed care view holds that disease management is a series of processes that (1) identify those members of managed health care plans who are at risk for chronic disease and (2) manage their care to avoid or delay onset of acute episodes."[106]

Eichert defines "disease management [as] the process of *managing the behaviors* of recipients, providers, and the system of healthcare delivery, across the continuum of care, based on the natural course of a disease. The goal is to optimize the effectiveness, efficiency, and quality of care. A disease management system will link the individual sectors of healthcare delivery through information systems designed to gather data, enhance communication, eliminate waste and duplication, and facilitate continuous learning and improvement."[107]

The Zitter Group also defines disease management as "a comprehensive, integrated approach to care and reimbursement based on the natural course of the disease, with treatment designed to address an illness with maximum effectiveness and efficiency."[108]

Because of the emphasis on managing behaviors, disease management appears to be most effective when focused on illnesses and injuries that have a high potential for self-management by the client or family.[109] In other words, the focus of disease management is to get the client to take responsibility for the routine care required by the condition and to be aware of red flags that might signal that medical attention is needed. By managing the disease himself or herself, the client has a greater investment in health maintenance and costs are controlled because use of medical services is reduced. As a result, disease management is also an important aspect of client/family empowerment.

DEVELOPING AND IMPLEMENTING A DISEASE MANAGEMENT PROGRAM

To have a disease management program, extensive research must be performed to define and measure what good outcomes are and the treatment protocols that are most likely to lead to them. These measurements include the following:

- utilization outcomes for all members enrolled in the [disease management program];
- patient satisfaction and perceptions of general health and well-being;
- specific clinical outcomes for each program.[110]

Thus, careful research, analysis of data, and planning are integral parts of the development of any disease management program. A six-step process to developing an effective disease management program is recommended.[111] These six steps include (1) identifying key processes for client care according to severity, (2) examining the current system of care from the client's perspective and modify it to be more user friendly, (3) using research to define appropriate systems of care, (4) comparing the current process to that which is identified as more appropriate through the research process, (5) modifying or creating new systems of care as needed, and (6) establishing an oversight committee to monitor success and make continuous improvements.

Ward and Rieve[112] have identified a number of steps for the case manager to follow in putting a disease management program into practice. These steps are summarized below along with some additional information:

1. Clients who are at risk must be identified using a system of risk assessment, risk profiles, and criteria created for the purpose. These risk profiles also categorize clients by severity based on symptoms presented and treatment required (e.g., at risk, stable, unstable, and complex). To be cost efficient, these profiles must strike a balance between identifying too many and identifying too few clients for potential disease state case management.
2. Clinical pathways with a full spectrum of planned therapeutic interventions appropriate to the severity level of the client's disease resulting in repeatable, predictable outcomes must be defined.
3. To implement the disease management care plan, the case manager must review the benefit package to which the client is entitled in order to identify eligibility for services and benefits exclusions/limitations and, when appropriate, to make recommendations for benefits exceptions.
4. Based on this, appropriate customized case management services must be developed and in place for use with the at-risk populations and the individuals who comprise them. This includes development and implementation of treatment plans with clinical providers and client self-care management initiatives, with monitoring and rewarding of compliant

behavior. Packaged financial reimbursement methodologies as incentives for providers for proactive care while reducing costs also need to be included.

5. Implementation of the disease management plan by obtaining the consent and agreement of all parties concerned, including the client/family, payer, physician, and other providers. The process of implementation also involves education of the parties involved, which may be done through in-person contact, nurse call-in lines, and multimedia information for clients developed especially for the purpose.
6. Follow-up services must be conducted to ensure compliance and to adjust the plan as needed according to the client's individual requirements. As disease management often involves long term, chronic conditions, follow-up services may also be lengthy. The purpose of long term monitoring is to prevent acute flare-ups.
7. Tracking of outcomes as a result of the disease management program must be an ongoing process to ensure that the program is modified appropriately to take into consideration improvements in medical technology and knowledge of disease states. This includes comprehensive data collection and reporting.
8. Pricing of disease management programs can be either on a capitated or a fee-for-service basis. Increasingly, these programs are negotiating risk sharing contracts.

Third-party payers may already have their own disease management programs established. It is then the responsibility of the case manager to become familiar with these programs and the information required to implement them. If the third-party payer does not have its own disease management programs already defined, the firm providing the service may wish to develop this information from statistics obtained both from case management outcomes and data profiling.

Every case management firm must have access to information on disease management that is constantly being updated. This information needs to be available to case managers when they begin working on cases as they are reviewing the medical information available in the file.

The role of the case manager in disease management programs is similar to that in regular case management. The involvement of the case manager begins with screening patients for ability to benefit from this type of program, coordination of care, monitoring the care across the continuum of the health care delivery system, and assisting with critical pathway compliance.

SUGGESTED READINGS

Kornowski R, Zeeli E, Averbuch M: Intensive home-care surveillance prevents hospitalization and improves morbidity rates among elderly patients with severe congestive heart failure, *Am Heart J* 129(4): 762-766, 1995.

Kozma CM: Defining actionable markets for disease state management, *Med Interface* 9(5):91-92, 1996.

Kozma CM: Disease state management programs: demonstrating success, *Med Interface* 9(9):88-89, 1996.

Lumsdon K: Disease management: the heat and headaches over retooling patient care create hard labor, *Hospitals Health Networks* 34-38, 42, April 1995.

Naylor M, Brooten D: Comprehensive discharge planning for the hospitalized elderly, *Ann Intern Med* 120:199-1006, 1994.

Petersen C: Disease state management: a new view of an old idea, *Managed Healthcare* 45-48, May 1995.

Schneider JK, Hornberger S and others: A medication discharge planning program, *Clin Nursing Res* 2(1): 41-53, 1993.

Sylvestri MF: Health care informatics: the key to successful disease management, *Med Interface* 9(5):94-96, 98-99, 1996.

Ward MD, Rieve J: Disease management: case management's return to patient-centered care, *J Care Management* 1(4):7-12, 1995.

References are found at the end of the book.

CHAPTER 26

ADDRESSING CROSS-CULTURAL ISSUES

A component that often arises in counseling and interviewing is how to bridge the gap between cultures when a client/family is a member of a minority group. Working with minorities will become a more significant component of case management if current predictions by the Department of Labor (USDOL) come true. According to the USDOL, "white males will make up only 15% of the increase in the workforce before 2000 and a third of all entrants into the labor force will be minorities."[113]

There are many issues that can be discussed in relationship to multiculturalism in case management practice, but this chapter touches only briefly on some areas of concern. The purpose of this chapter is to encourage the case manager to consider the client's point of view when working with minority groups or individuals from a different culture. As many cultures have no case manager-type role and may be used to a very different type of health care system, one of the first steps for the case manager is to explain his or her role and the American health care system.[114]

When one thinks of minority groups, African Americans, Hispanics, Native Americans, Indochinese refugees, and other foreign-born individuals usually come to mind. However, there are other groups with their own distinct cultures, such as deaf persons who use American Sign Language and certain religious groups (e.g., Jehovah's Witnesses, Christian Scientists, Amish, Mennonites, Muslims, Hindus), who eschew some of the trappings of American culture, Western medicine, and modern life. In some cases, it is not evident that an individual is a member of a minority group that may affect medical decisions.

LANGUAGE BARRIERS

Language barriers are one cross-cultural issue that is readily evident. If the case manager and the client do not speak the same language, communication is difficult or impossible. Obtaining the services of an interpreter is the most obvious solution. When resources are limited, case managers are sometimes reluctant to request authorization for payment of the services of a professional interpreter. Often, the client's family members offer to interpret at no cost, and the case manager is tempted to let them do it. Using family members as interpreters does have the advantage of saving money, but it can create difficulties because family members are not objective observers. They may have some personal, cultural, financial, or emotional stake in the proceedings and may choose to censor or misrepresent what the case manager, the client, and others are saying for their own benefit. Family members also may not be as proficient in the two languages as they claim to be, resulting in inadequate translation of some concepts. This is especially true about technical terminology, such as medical nomenclature.

Professional interpreters, on the other hand, may be certified for medical or legal work, which indicates that they have the expertise to translate technical terminology and have a basic level of skill in both languages. They also tend to be more objective than family members. Professional interpreters can be obtained through language banks in many of the larger urban areas of the country. They may also be available through community centers that serve people who come from the same country or speak the same language (e.g., community centers for the deaf, Hispanics, or Southeast Asians).

The use of interpreters is not just confined to conversations and meetings. Case managers often find that it is helpful to have written materials translated. The written instructions given to clients when they leave an inpatient or residential facility should be translated if the client or caregivers cannot read them in English. Notices from the carrier or other sources regarding noncoverage of treatments or procedures should certainly be translated so that there are no misunderstandings.

DIFFERENCES IN WORLDVIEWS AMONG CULTURES

Being able to deal with cross-cultural issues goes far beyond being able to translate languages. It involves an appreciation that the client/family may have a very different worldview than the case manager and medical providers. One often hears the cliché that "something is lost in translation." That "something" is often the cultural values of the person whose words are being translated. In addition, literal translations of some concepts may be quite different from what the person intended to communicate. For example, the term "persistent vegetative state" might be translated as "plant" in Chinese.

Another important concept is that some clients are bilingual, bicultural, or both.[115] This means that some individuals may speak a different language, but they have largely absorbed the values of the American culture. Others may speak fluent English but may adhere to the cultural values of another country, a religion, or other minority group within this country. Yet others have limited familiarity with either English or the American culture. The important thing to remember is that acculturation and assimilation occur on a continuum.[116]

In some cultures, disabilities and certain illnesses are viewed with shame, and the person with less than perfect health is blamed for the condition and may be considered less valuable as a human being. (For example, some religions, such as Hinduism, believe that afflictions in this life are a product of working out negative karma from a past life.) Families in some cultures may believe that they must adopt what most American health care professionals would regard as an overprotective stance toward the client, thus depriving him or her of the independence needed for an optimal recovery.

Immigrants from Communist and former Soviet bloc nations may not have a clear understanding of how a capitalistic society works. This will affect them both vocationally and as consumers of medical goods and services.

DEVELOPING TRUST WITH CLIENTS FROM DIFFERENT CULTURES

Although there are many minority groups in this country, the largest are African American and Hispanic. It has been noted that "in 1985, the U.S. population totaled 238 million; 12

percent were African American, 5.8 percent Hispanic, 1.6 percent Asian, 0.6 percent [Native American] and 80 percent Anglo American. . . . By the year 2020 demographers predict that Anglo Americans will [only] account for 70 percent of the total U.S. population."[117] However, there is a larger percentage of African Americans with disabilities and other health-related problems; 13.4% of African Americans have disabilities versus 8.4% of Anglo Americans.[118]

In working with both African American and Hispanic populations, case managers have to guard against the perpetuation of long-standing racial and ethnic stereotypes. According to Feist-Price and Ford-Harris, "Many African American clients present five barriers in counseling: (1) a negative attitude towards counseling; (2) the expectation of therapeutic failure; (3) defensiveness and fear of self-disclosure because of identification with societal stereotypes of males being super masculine and females as super strong . . . ; (4) feelings of discomfort during counseling; and (5) the counselor's own discomfort in working with African American clients."[119]

Overcoming these obstacles requires, as a baseline, adopting Rogers' notion of "unconditional positive regard"[120] in order to develop trust and provide African American clients with positive but realistic information about their options and potential. Case managers also need to learn to identify what it is like to be a minority in the American culture, especially a minority that is associated with many negative stereotypes.

Basic Premises for Working With Diverse Populations

Addressing all the issues related to case management of African Americans and Hispanics is beyond the scope of this book. Case managers who work with diverse populations should avail themselves of the many workshops, training opportunities, and literature available on this subject as the American population becomes increasingly multicultural. In working with members of other cultures, the case manager must remember some basic premises:

- *Avoid ethnocentrism and religious chauvinism.* Ethnocentrism is the belief that one's own culture is the most valid and correct. Even though a case manager may prefer the way things are done in his or her own culture, he or she needs to be able to objectively view other cultures and religions as equally valid for those who are part of them. Unless the practices of another culture or religion are clearly detrimental to the medical or personal well-being of the client, they must be accepted and honored. This sounds reasonable in theory, but in real life, it is often extremely nebulous and subject to the personal prejudices of the case manager, medical providers, and the legal system. A number of legal battles have been fought over parents' rights to deprive minor children of needed medical treatment that goes against their religion. Recently, the desire for physician-performed female circumcision by parents of Muslim girls has been a subject of considerable controversy.
- *Remember that "Culture is a learned, shared, and symbolically transmitted design for living."*[121] This means that all members of a minority group have common values that bind them in a broad sense, but individual members of the same culture may not necessarily share the same viewpoint on some specific things. All cultures have factions within them that cause individual members of the culture to differ sharply on certain matters.

Cultural values are often transmitted through language, legends, myths, and metaphors. The case manager must learn the terms that are used to convey cultural values but may not be able to rely on one member of a cultural group to speak for all members of the group on certain matters.

Likewise, members of some cultures may disagree with certain values of their culture but are unwilling to go against them because there is considerable social pressure within the group to conform. The case manager may be able to address this issue by giving the client/family strong assurances about right-to-privacy and confidentiality issues.

- *Examine your own cultural relativism issues.* The case manager needs to try to understand people's beliefs from the point of view of their culture. Even though the case manager does not share the same beliefs as the client, he or she still needs to respect them if the belief systems are not refutable or strongly counter to the client's best interests. This means working within the belief system to effect positive outcomes. For example, the client's religion may encourage her to believe that she is to blame for her illness and that it is a curse for some wrongdoing, or bad karma, on her part. The case manager may not be able to refute this belief but can show the client that she can take steps to minimize the effects of the illness even though it is destiny and has to be accepted.

  Some of the ways other cultures differ from modern American life are related to how people regard nature, time, and each other. For example, many cultures do not feel the time pressures that are endemic in American life. People from those cultures may see no need for rapid decision making or rapid transitions in life and may be lax about keeping appointments and being on time. Likewise, some cultures do not place emphasis on the individual but rather on the group. At times, this even extends to blurred boundaries regarding personal property and individual rights. For example, in some cultures, adults are still expected to obey their parents and to make decisions that the group regards as important but may not necessarily be in the best interests of the individual.
- *Recognize the role of the family.* Families of individuals from other cultures often tend to be large and extended, with several generations living in the same household. Some cultures appear to be male dominated on the surface, but in reality, the women may be responsible for decision making even though this is subtle and unobtrusive.[122] Therefore, it may not be helpful to face down the authority of male family members but to communicate with responsible and influential females who appear to have matriarchal roles.
- *Remember that all clients are entitled to culture-sensitive care.* The value system that most mainstream Americans have "about controlling nature, the value of human life, [only having one life to live], the belief in a biophysical reality all underlie a narrow perspective on health and illness."[123] Most people do not find it easy to transcend their belief systems to truly work within another culture.
  - *Illness-disease beliefs.* Case managers need to find out from the client what his or her beliefs are about the cause, definition, and cure of the condition in question.

The answer to these questions may lie in spiritual beliefs rather than in medical science as most Americans understand it.

- *Standard American medical practice versus folk medicine.* For some clients to recover, it may be necessary to combine these two systems. It has been noted that "an estimated 70% to 90% of all self-recognized episodes of sickness are managed exclusively outside the perimeter of the formal healthcare system."[124] Also, there is increasing acceptance among mainstream Americans of the value of such non-Western remedies as herbal treatments, homeopathy, and acupuncture.
- *Knowledge, mutual respect, and negotiation.* The client and case manager must talk about cultural issues to gain mutual understanding and to negotiate a plan of action that respects all viewpoints. Sometimes, considerable time in counseling sessions has to be devoted to this, and the case manager may have to research other cultures because the members of the culture may take some of their beliefs so much for granted that they are not able to articulate the difference between their values and those of the case manager.

GOAL IN A CROSS-CULTURAL ENVIRONMENT

Thus, the goal of case management in a cross-cultural environment is to somehow bridge the gap in knowledge and expectations to achieve a treatment plan that addresses the expectations of the client's culture and the systems and operations of the medical establishment. This is not an easy process because it calls for openmindedness on the part of the case manager and a willingness to learn and develop unorthodox and creative solutions to problems and issues. All of a case manager's interviewing, active listening, and counseling skills and creativity come into play as well as his or her medical expertise. The case manager's personal awareness of his or her own cultural background, values, and systems is essential in coming to an understanding of the client's cultural context.

SUGGESTED READINGS

Alston RJ, Bell TJ, Feist-Price S: Racial identity and African Americans with disabilities: theoretical and practical considerations, *J Rehab* 62(2):11-15, 1996.

American Health Consultants: Changes in U.S. demographics force CMs to address patients' cultural diversity, *Case Management Advisor* 5(11):145-150, 1994.

Geiger D: *Transcultural nursing: assessment and intervention,* ed 2, St. Louis, 1995, Mosby.

Helms JE: *Black and white racial identity: theory, research, and practice,* New York, 1990, Greenwood Press.

Leal-Idrogo A: Further thoughts on "The use of interpreters and translators in delivery of rehabilitation services," *J Rehab* 61(2):21-23, 1995.

Ong WMA: *Asian American cultural dimensions in rehabilitation counseling,* San Diego, Calif, 1993, Diego State University, Rehabilitation Cultural Diversity Initiative.

Randall DE: *Strategies for working with culturally diverse communities and clients,* Washington, DC, 1989, Association for the Care of Children's Health.

Smart JF, Smart DW: The rehabilitation of Hispanics experiencing acculturative stress: implications for practice, *J Rehab* 61(2):14-20, 1994.

Smart JF, Smart DW: The use of translators/interpreters in rehabilitation, *J Rehab* 61(2):14-20, 1995.

Spector RE: *Cultural diversity in health and illness,* ed 3, East Norwalk, Conn, 1991, Appleton & Lange.

References are found at the end of the book.

CHAPTER 27

FUTURE OF CASE MANAGEMENT

It is indeed dangerous in these times of change and evolution in health care to be discussing the future of a dynamic program such as case management. There are many forces in place, from integrated delivery systems to capitated contracting to data report cards, that will, no doubt, affect how case management adapts. All of these developments and more will affect how case management functions in the future.

Nevertheless, there have been trends in case management leading to some reasonable assumptions on how case management will evolve in light of the health care delivery and insurance system changes. A description of how it appears that case management will change in several key areas is given in the following sections.

ROLE OF THE CLIENT

In health care generally, the client or patient has been viewed as a passive participant in the health care process. The physician would tell the patient what to do, what the treatment plan was, and how things were going to progress. In this country, most patients historically accepted the physician's decision and followed orders.

For many reasons, that scenario has changed for the good. Providers and health plans now view clients as consumers of health care who must be courted. Consumers are now being surveyed for their satisfaction levels, provided health education on topics relevant to their condition, and educated on the health care system. The goal is for consumers or clients to become more involved in their own health care.

Some consumers have become more assertive about their health care needs. Disability rights groups, most notably AIDS advocacy groups, have become more vocal in the expression of their expectations and their demands from health care systems and providers for the treatment of their conditions. The AIDS crisis resulted in providers dealing with more informed consumers who, at times, knew more than providers about their condition and available treatment options. Case managers will need to be ready to deal with consumers who are informed, assertive, and clear about their expectations. This type of client should actually be easier to work with than more passive clients who want the case manager to make decisions for them.

Case management is taking that scenario a step further by allowing clients to become the key decision makers in their own health care. The case manager's role is to present the options, the consequences of those options, and the implementation activities for each of the options. It is then up to the client, with whomever he or she chooses to assist in the decision-making process, to decide how the case will proceed. The client may involve the family, significant other, trusted friend or advisor, or the attending physician, or any combination of these, in the decision. The client may ask the case manager to conduct further research or provide more information about the options presented. It will then be the responsibility of the case manager to inform, coordinate, and implement the decision the client makes. This may be very difficult for some case managers who, as trained health care providers, may think the decision being made is not the best one for the client in the long run. In any event, case managers must shift to this kind of role and, consequently, will need to improve on the ability to make convincing presentations of the available options and choices for clients and become more comfortable with choices with which they disagree.

GOALS OF INTERVENTION

Clearly, the reason for the birth of case management was cost containment. Health plans, employers, and other purchasers of case management services made their decision to use such services based on the need to save money and control costs (see Chapter 1 for further discussion). Case management firms responded by creating sound methodologies to document cost savings and data reports to profile the results. Case managers negotiated discounted rates with providers and vendors, arranged for prompt exchange of expensive inpatient settings with less costly levels of care, and monitored the necessity of continued outpatient and ancillary services. For workers' compensation and LTD cases, the speed with which the case manager was able to establish medical stability, render an employability statement, or return the client to work was the key to satisfied referral sources. Outcomes measurement for case management was entirely focused on the amount of cost savings, and referral sources often made their referral decisions based on the amount of cost savings promised or demonstrated.

The focus on cost containment is very understandable in the historical context of health insurance costs escalating at double digit annual inflation rates. Also, health plans were typically working within a fee-for-service or discounted fee-for-service environment, so that cost containment was the key focus. Benefit plans were desperate to slow the skyrocketing costs of health care, and case management addressed the most expensive cases.

As previously discussed, capitated contracts with provider groups and integrated delivery systems (IDS) are becoming more commonplace. As a result of these new reimbursement methodologies, case management intervention and outcomes measurement will need to change accordingly. If the IDS, for example, is capitated for certain services, the plan and the case manager no longer need to focus on controlling costs, as the financial arrangement has taken care of the financial risk. The health plan, through the case manager, needs to now focus on the quality and access to appropriate care. New methodologies and strategies for assessing appropriate quality and access need to be developed. Data profiling and analysis, as well as individual case review, can be done to assess these areas, but there also need to be practice standards, pathways, or criteria available with which to compare the data.

Referral sources and case management firms will need to develop new outcomes measurements as a result of this new focus on quality and access. Case managers will also need to become more sophisticated with statistical analysis and more familiar with standards and pathways. Case management intervention will probably be most appropriate when a patient has "fallen off" the designated clinical pathway. Case managers may also need to advocate for clients when they have not received enough care from the health care delivery system. These are new roles for case managers, and cost containment can no longer be the single most important element in measuring outcomes. Such factors as consumer satisfaction, compliance with practice standards, involvement with improvement projects, and compliance with access standards may well become the measurement of case management success in the future.

TIMING OF INTERVENTION

Case management began in the workers' compensation sector when claims managers recognized long-term, chronic cases that needed some type of intervention to better control costs. This occurred after high claims costs were incurred along with months of **time-loss.** In the health insurance sector, case management was initially identified at the time of admission to a hospital. Cases were screened not only for the appropriateness of the admission but also for their potential for case management intervention.

These methods resulted in being too late in the process to be as effective as possible. It has been routinely asserted that the earlier case management intervenes, the better the outcomes.[125] As a result of this and in an effort to be more competitive, health plans and systems have developed earlier methods of identifying clients for case management intervention. For workers' compensation, carriers and employers have set up better systems for immediate identification of on-the-job injuries so that case management can intervene within hours of the injury. This not only helps to improve on the effectiveness of case management, but it also helps to reduce litigation, improve relations with the employer, and return the injured worker to work or medical stability or both. In the health insurance arena, health plans have begun to screen new consumers at the time of enrollment to detect any need for case management intervention. This strategy gets to the consumer before any health care services have even been accessed. It anticipates the needs and assesses the risk of these new consumers so that the case manager can help the new consumer through the new health care delivery system.

FOCUS OF INTERVENTION

Because historically the focus of case management was cost containment and the intervention occurred when the client reached the hospital, the focus of case management was to discharge the patient to a safe, less costly, lower level of care. Some referral sources saw case management as an intensive discharge planning activity, so that once the client was discharged from the hospital with appropriate home care negotiated and coordinated, there was no further need for case management intervention. This is a short-sighted view of the possibilities of the function and role of case management and obviously assumes the dominance of the cost-containment goal.

Increasingly, case management is seen as necessary across the continuum of care, regardless of the setting or the case acuity level. Certainly, the intensity of case management activity varies depending on the setting and demands of care, but the value of case management is seen beyond the walls of a hospital. Consumer education about health care issues and delivery system idiosyncrasies is becoming an essential function for case managers. Monitoring not only the appropriateness of use but the quality of ancillary service providers is also a new area for case managers. Cases may stay open longer for ongoing monitoring, and the acuity levels of caseloads may decrease if case management interventions beyond inpatient hospitalizations are deemed appropriate by the health plan. Case managers may be able to develop more ongoing relationships with the clients they work with, but the caution here is that dependency on the part of the client may develop. The case manager must continue to be clear in his or her role with the client, so the client continues to feel empowered and responsible for his or her own health care. The function of the case manager will evolve from cost controller to educator, integrator, supporter, and ongoing continuum of care coordinator.

ROLE OF THE HEALTH CARE SYSTEM

When case management began years ago, the providers typically viewed case managers as unnecessary interventionists sent by the insurance carrier to check up on them. There was confusion about what exactly the case managers were trying to accomplish. Some saw case managers as threats, others saw them as spies of the insurance company, and still others saw them as duplicating services. Clearly, case managers were viewed as external, third-party representatives with uncertain goals.

Case management concepts and goals have become more commonplace. In fact, some health care systems have employed their own case managers to assist the clients in their facilities and clinics. Savvy health care providers, especially home health and home infusion providers, see case managers as a way to channel clients to their services. Case managers are viewed increasingly as essential members of the treatment team, and, as IDSs grow in size (see Chapter 3 for further discussion), case managers may become the cement to the system, or what can be called "system integrators." Not only will case managers continue in their role as evaluators, coordinators, and implementors, but they are now becoming the resource for consumers who need to make their way through an ever more confusing health care delivery system maze.

PROVIDER RELATIONS

As discussed previously, case managers have become more commonly accepted by providers, so that the initial antagonistic, distrustful relationships of the past are disappearing.[126] Providers have seen the need for a variety of managed care techniques and strategies. Case management is one of the more positive programs employed by managed care organizations. Consequently, providers are seeing the value of the case manager's role, including information on benefit plan provisions, exclusions, and limitations, along with exceptions to these issues. Providers have also begun to see case managers as opportunities to receive more referrals and, thus, more revenues. The relationship between case managers and providers has included information sharing and price negotiations. Providers have started to see that case managers are not merely the unthinking agents of the insurance carrier or health plan but, rather, fulfill the role of communicator and advocate when necessary.

As health plans and the IDS phenomenon evolve with more capitated contracts in place, providers and case managers will see changes in their relationships. Case managers will need to work even more collaboratively with providers to address such issues as quality of care and access standards. Case managers can offer assistance for working with more difficult clients who do not follow the normal course of treatment or the defined disease management plan. Statistical analysis of aggregate patters of care/treatment may need to be conducted jointly between providers and case managers to determine the areas in need of improvement. Once there is agreement on the key issues, case managers and providers may need to work together to develop, implement, and monitor improvement plans. Case managers may well become the critical professionals for making the much discussed system integration truly work for providers as well as for consumers. All of this points to an even more positive and valued relationship between case managers and providers.

BILLING

Historically, case managers have billed on an hourly, fee-for-service basis, like other health care providers. There has been competition based on hourly rates. For example, some case management firms have differentiated rates for professional time versus travel/wait time. There has been some discounting of hourly rates based on volume of anticipated cases, yet the primary pricing structure has been historically based on hourly reimbursement. There have been some trends to have case management pricing based on case rates. That is, based on the type of case (e.g., head injury), the case management firm would receive a set fee amount regardless of the number of hours spent on the case. The case rate methodology has also been used for certain kinds of activities. For example, in workers' compensation cases, case managers have been paid a set amount of money for rehabilitation plan development or for job search assistance. These strategies have been used by referral sources as ways to better control the amount of case management activity authorized and expended.

Because much of health care is moving toward capitation pricing, so is case management. Health plans are including case management services at a set capitated rate based on a per member per month (PMPM) price. Whether the plan provides this internally or externally, plans are setting the amount of case management resources to be used on a fixed capitated rate. Again, like other health care providers under this new reimbursement methodology, case management firms face difficult decisions, sometimes presenting ethical dilemmas, such as what kinds of cases are selected for intervention, how long case management continues, what is the most effective service delivery approach (on-site versus telephonic), and what are the performance expectations of case management. The role of the professional case manager will need to be better delineated. One idea is to create functions for case management assistants to provide paraprofessional support.

These kinds of actions can actually improve on the efficiency and outcome of the case management process. However, the challenge under capitation is to be able to continue to deliver high-quality services while not being overly influenced by the reimbursement methodology, which encourages a case manager to limit the amount of intervention.[127,128] Assistance from actuaries or other professionals may be helpful while entertaining these kinds of contracts. There may even be reinsurance coverage available in the future for case management firms that enter into capitated contracts. Assessing and controlling the risk of capitated contracts will be essential for all health care providers, including case management providers.

Besides capitation, another trend in billing is the risk corridor concept. This works similarly to capitation because there is a range of money (e.g., a retainer) or billable hours that is paid monthly, quarterly, or annually. If services involve fewer than the range of hours or dollars in the risk corridor, the case management company is usually required to pay back the extra funds. This repayment usually takes place quarterly or annually. If it is necessary for the case manager to go over the maximum number of hours in the risk corridor, it is necessary to request special approval from the customer. Because the customer is interested in controlling costs, it is usually necessary to have good justification for asking for more money or hours.

With this risk corridor concept, there is an incentive for the case management firm to stay at the lower end of the risk corridor range because they are allowed to keep the additional funds in the risk corridor if they do not use all of them. Because the number of hours used tends to vary from month to month, the case management firm will also maintain a steady cash flow during the times (summer and holidays) when fewer services are provided. Also, it is advantageous to the customer because case managers will not be calling frequently to request additional authorizations, and the case manager will have an incentive to be parsimonious with billable hours and expenses.

REFERRAL SOURCE RELATIONS

Because case management is a service, the selling process tends to be based on the relationship established between the referral source and the case management provider. Referral sources have become somewhat distrustful of case management as a whole because of a variety of factors, such as overselling of the program, overbilling, lack of adequate data reporting, overstatement of the cost savings, tremendous variation in case management models, and misunderstandings about the goals and functions of case management. In some instances, referral sources view case management as a necessary evil that must be regretfully implemented. As a result, some case management firms continue in their role as a vendor of services that are widely available and undistinguished.

To survive in an increasingly competitive environment, case management firms will need to move beyond the vendor mentality. This will require increased business sophistication and improved customer relationship skills. Case management firms should look at the long-term relationship with referral sources, which takes time, attention, and good planning to be successful. Rather than being merely a vendor of services, case management firms can establish themselves as trusted advisors, even partners, with referral sources.

Referral sources want to be treated as more than simply a revenue source. Their needs and wants need to be explored in addition to their long-term goals and plans for how they wish to operate in the future. Case management firms are well poised to assist referral sources in such areas as benefit plan design, delivery system integration and functioning, customer satisfaction, improvement projects, quality of care issues, access to compliance standards, and provider relations.

Responsive, knowledgeable, and honest concern is a key ingredient that case management firms can demonstrate to referral sources. Examples of this might include sharing of articles on relevant topics, conducting seminars or symposiums for referral sources on timely issues, providing research at no charge, and visiting customers routinely to discuss how to improve on the case management program. Referral sources do not want to feel

BOX 27-1

OTHER IMPLICATIONS FOR THE FUTURE OF CASE MANAGEMENT

- *Disease management and population management* will be more important in the years to come. (For more detailed information, refer to Chapter 24 on disease management.) In the past, case managers have worked mostly with individual patients. In the future, they will work more and more with aggregate populations to manage large numbers of patients in a manner that is more cost efficient than providing services to individuals.
- *Clinical specialization.* Historically, most case managers tended to be generalists, but the trend toward greater clinical specialization of case managers has been gaining momentum in the last 10 years or so and will increase as time goes on. Because of the trend toward disease management and population management, case managers will be expected to have a higher level of clinical expertise with the diseases and populations with which they work.
- *Quantifying* ***outcomes management*** *(statistical analysis).* In conjunction with the disease management of populations, there will be more emphasis placed on statistical analysis of aggregate groups in relation to their health outcomes, cost outcomes, and customer satisfaction. Similarly, data will be analyzed to profile providers in terms of health and cost outcomes. This type of focus is another indication of the trend toward moving away from subjective work with individual clients to objective analysis of aggregate populations.
- *Changes in education of registered nurses and other professionals to support process of case management.* Thus far, most training in case management has occurred on the job or in workshops sponsored by various organizations of case managers. Currently, the trend is toward academic involvement in the training of case managers through colleges and universities for bachelor's and master's degree programs.[129] Academia is also involved in research to statistically validate the process of case management and the outcomes that result from it. Although case management has traditionally been a very practical discipline, the trend is toward making it more theoretical and academic.
- *Preventive case management.* Since its inception, case management has been mostly a crisis-oriented approach that occurred following an injury or illness. Now, there is a trend toward using it as a preventive tool in disease management and population management. Case managers are now working in occupational health and safety programs as well.
- *Mediation.* Case managers are now participating in formal mediation and conflict resolution processes because they can supply valuable information to settle conflicts more equitably without going to court. This is particularly true in regard to life care planning.[130] By participating in formal mediation, case managers can help prevent litigation and manage limited available funds. Following the award of funds, case managers can also assist with the management of funding to ensure that money is allocated where it is most needed.

unimportant or neglected, as this is one of the primary reasons for any customer to discontinue doing business. Referral sources want to feel that their business, contracts, and clients are important to the case management provider. How a case management firm goes about establishing itself as a valued ally will depend on the corporate culture and the customer base for each individual firm. Yet the need to become more than just a vendor and more like a partner is essential for the future of case management. Box 27-1 describes likely future trends in case management.

SUMMARY

At present, case management is one of the fastest growing medically related professions in the United States. Because there is ever increasing pressure to contain medical costs and medical science is progressing so rapidly, case management has been undergoing rapid and dramatic changes over the last 10 years. As these health care reform and cost-containment trends do not seem to be abating, the progress of case management will continue to move at the speed of light well into the next century. Although growth is always stressful to some extent, these changes are also exciting and challenging because they are improving the professionalism of case management and, therefore, helping to garner more respect for the profession as a whole.

SUGGESTED READINGS

Lemire ET: Community-based health reform: a case management model for consumer self-determination, *J Care Management* 2(3):9-11, 14, 16, 18, 21-22, 24, 26, 1996.

Murer M: Managed care trends: case management challenges in integrated health systems, *Continuing Care* 15(4):14, 30, 1996.

Reich P: Capitation and ethics, *Med Interface* 9(9):16, 1996.

Romaine DS: Case management challenges, present and future, *Continuing Care* 14(1):24-31, 1995.

References are found at the end of the book.

APPENDIXES

APPENDIX 1
EXAMPLES OF CRITERIA

CONTENTS

BOX A1-1

CASE MANAGEMENT PRENOTIFICATION LIST

Admission of more than 10 days
Cancer
Cerebrovascular accident/stroke (CVA)
Chemical dependency—*see* Psychiatric and chemical dependency
Chronic respiratory disease
Congenital defects
Congenital heart disease
Diabetes
HIV disease
Ischemic heart disease/peripheral vascular disease
Neonatal complications
Neurodegenerative disorders (multiple sclerosis, amyotrophic lateral sclerosis, muscular dystrophy)
Organ transplant
Pregnancy, complications of
Psychiatric and chemical dependency
Spinal cord injury
Trauma (multiple trauma, head injury)

BOX A1-2

INFORMATION FROM INTAKE

Admitting diagnosis
Primary care physician—name and telephone number
Approximate length of stay
Need for skilled nursing facility, durable medical equipment (DME), or home health services for hospice or other outpatient service needs
Name and telephone number of discharge planner.
Care conference—when, who

BOX A1-3

INFORMATION FROM HEALTH CARE COORDINATORS

Alternative Setting for Treatment: Long-Term, Acute Care, Specialty Centers

Home health care, hospice care, or public health involvement before this admission—name
Rehabilitation—goals, inpatient, outpatient, home
Care conference—contact
Psychosocial issues—primary caregiver in home, transportation, patient reliability, patient compliance
Other medical problems
Targeted discharge date
Discharge plan—long-term care, specialty center, home health care, hospice, skilled nursing facility
Durable medical equipment needs—oxygen, medical supplies

BOX A1-4

CLINICAL SCREENING CRITERIA

1 ADMISSION OF MORE THAN 10 DAYS

Immediate Referral to Case Management Screening

Any admission longer than 10 days

Health Information to Obtain

Diagnosis on admission
Present condition—complications
Current treatment plans—medications, treatments, latest laboratory work
Clinical coordinator's name and number/ social worker's name and number

2 CANCER

Immediate Referral to Case Management Screening

Bone marrow transplant
Peripheral stem cell transplants (PSCT)
Oat cell lung cancer
Pancreatic cancer
Liver cancer
Glioblastoma
Astrocytoma
Metastatic cancer
Esophageal/laryngeal cancer
Leukemia
Pediatric oncology

Health Information to Obtain

Surgical or medical admission
Stage of treatment
Prognosis
Medical stage of disease
Other medications required—e.g., antiemetics
Pain management issues
Other treatment modalities

3 CEREBROVASCULAR ACCIDENT (CVA)

Immediate Referral to Case Management Screening

CVA with underlying medical issues—history of bypass surgery, diabetes, deep vein thrombosis (DVT), peripheral vascular disease
CVA with greater than 2 weeks estimated length of stay in rehabilitation
CVA needing home care, purchase of large durable medical supplies, and/or an alternative placement

Health Information to Obtain

Cognitive ability
Nutritional status
Long-term effects, residual deficits
Length of recovery time
Rehabilitation potential
Current treatment plan
Underlying disease process
Prognosis

4 CHRONIC RESPIRATORY DISEASE

Immediate Referral to Case Management Screening

Hypoxemia
Hypercapnia
Severe asthmatic or emphysema diagnosis—two or more ER or hospital admissions per year
Chronic obstructive pulmonary disease (COPD)—two or more admissions per year
Cystic fibrosis
Any admission to an intensive care unit (ICU) with respiratory failure

Health Information to Obtain

Medications
Progression of disease
Functional limitations

5 CONGENITAL HEART DISEASE

Immediate Referral to Case Management Screening

Tetralogy of Fallot
Truncus arteriosus
Transposition of the great vessels
Atrial septal defect (ASD)
Congential heart defect
Dextrocardia
Asplenia

Continued

BOX A1-4

CLINICAL SCREENING CRITERIA—cont'd

5 CONGENITAL HEART DISEASE—cont'd

Ventral septal defect (VSD)
Requests for home oxygen for children under 18 years

Health Information to Obtain

Cardiopulmonary complications—shortness of breath, oxygen needs
Neurocognitive complications
Medications
Laboratory values—ammonia levels, ejection fraction
Pretransplant
Prenatal complications—chemical dependency, medications

6 DIABETES

Immediate Referral to Case Management Screening

Insulin-dependent diabetes—new onset
Diabetic coma
Diabetic ketoacidosis
Juvenile diabetes
Cellulitis, osteomyelitis
Pregnancy-induced diabetes
ER visit or admission for diabetic control

Health Information to Obtain

Formal diabetic education
Complications—hyperglycemia, hypoglycemia, dehydration
Neurologic status, periods of confusion, neuropathies
Renal complications—high BUN, creatinine
Integumentary status—decubitus ulcers or areas requiring debridement
Gastrointestinal symptoms—nausea, vomiting, diarrhea pain, cramping
Latest laboratory work—glyconated hemoglobin, chemistry
Recent changes in medication regimen—insulin, oral insulin, implantable devices
Other medical conditions

7 HIV/AIDS

Immediate Referral to Case Management Screening

HIV positive

Health Information to Obtain

Respiratory complications—*Pneumocystis carinii* pneumonia, shortness of breath
Gastrointestinal complications—nausea and vomiting, diarrhea, dehydration/hypovolemia, wasting
Neurologic complications—AIDS dementia/confusion, complications from peripheral neuropathies
Integumentary complications—Kaposi's sarcoma, herpes, fungal infections
Visual complications
Current laboratory values
Medication regimen

8 ISCHEMIC HEART DISEASE

Immediate Referral to Case Management Screening

Two or more cardiac admissions in last 3 months
Length of stay greater than 10 days

Health Information to Obtain

Medication
Transplant potential
Angina at rest
Previous cardiac procedures
Recent testing—treadmill, catheterization
What is the ejection fraction?
Other complicating conditions

9 NEONATAL COMPLICATIONS

Immediate Referral to Case Management Screening

Extreme prematurity—less than 32 weeks gestation
Compromised respiratory status requiring prolonged treatment
Congential defects—long-term intervention or a component of a syndrome

BOX A1-4

CLINICAL SCREENING CRITERIA—cont'd

9 NEONATAL COMPLICATIONS—cont'd

Health Information to Obtain

Weeks gestation
Birth weight, Apgar score
Respiratory status
Cardiac status
Nutritional status—rate of feeding, nippling, gavage feeding
Mother's prenatal care
Community resources involved
Home situation—psychosocial issues

10 NEURODEGENERATIVE DISORDERS

Immediate Referral to Case Management Screening

Multiple sclerosis
Guillian-Barré syndrome
Cerebral palsy
Muscular dystrophy
Amyotrophic lateral sclerosis (ALS)

Health Information to Obtain

Progression of disease
Neurologist—name
Medications specific to diagnosis
Current treatment plan

11 ORGAN TRANSPLANT

Immediate Referral to Case Management Screening

Cardiac transplant
Cardiac/lung transplant
Liver transplant
Transplant involving two or more organs

Health Information to Obtain

Patient compliance with current treatment
Other chronic illness or disease process
Special assistive devices

12 PREGNANCIES

Immediate Referral to Case Management Screening

Two or more ER or outpatient hospital visits
Medical complications—three or more fetuses, hyperemesis gravidarum, total placenta abruptio, premature rupture of membranes (PROM), abdominal or cervical surgery during pregnancy, autoimmune disease
HELLP syndrome (hemolysis, elevated liver enzymes, low platelets)
Diethylstilbestrol (DES) exposure
Psychosocial issues—domestic violence, chemical dependency, delayed or no prenatal care

Potential Case Management Referral

Medical complications—twin gestations, cervical changes, hypertension (PIH), gestational diabetes, psychiatric signs and symptoms
History of preterm labor and/or birth
Bleeding—placenta previa, partial placenta abruptio
Oligohydramnio, polyhydramnios, intrauterine growth retardation (IUGR)

Health Information to Obtain

Bleeding after 12th week
Uterine irritability or contractions—frequency
If PROM present, when did it occur?
History of pyelonephritis, current diagnosis of beta-streptococcal infection, sexually transmitted disease (STD), uterine anomaly (e.g., fibroids)
Family history of diabetes
Name of primary care provider if different from admitting provider
Estimated date of confinement (EDC)

13 PSYCHIATRIC AND CHEMICAL DEPENDENCY

Immediate Referral to Case Management Screening

Evaluation for psychiatric partial hospitalization in lieu of inpatient stay

Continued

BOX A1-4

CLINICAL SCREENING CRITERIA—cont'd

13 PSYCHIATRIC AND CHEMICAL DEPENDENCY—cont'd

Evidence of major organ involvement related to chemical dependency issues
Evidence of chronic and repeated psychiatric or chemical dependency issues

Health Information to Obtain

Signs and symptoms on admission—affect, mood, physical presentation, suicidal/homicidal ideation, level of cooperativeness, hallucinations, delusional-paranoid
Chemical dependency—severity of detoxification, medical hospital or acute care chemical dependency facility
Precipitating event(s)
Psychiatric/chemical dependency history
Treatment history (inpatient/outpatient)
Current and past medical issues relevant to current condition
Current and past psychiatric medications
Placement in appropriate treatment—inpatient versus partial hospitalization
Behavior problems that could be attributed to a medical disorder, but behavior is to be addressed in a psychiatric setting—metabolic disorders, organic brain syndrome (OBS)
Psychosocial issues—support systems, family issues, social and extended treatment support systems
Discharge plans—placement, work

14 SPINAL CORD INJURY

Immediate Referral to Case Management Screening

Quadriplegia—new onset
Paraplegia—new onset
Existing paraplegia with complications

Health Information to Obtain

Medical history
Integumentary complications—history of decubiti, wounds, history of grafting
Urinary system complications
Bowel program
Cardiopulmonary complications
Potential access barriers

15 TRAUMA

Immediate Referral to Case Management Screening

Multiple fractures
Traumatic brain injury (TBI)—moderate or severe

Health Information to Obtain

Neurologic complications—current residual deficits, spinal cord involvement
Cognitive functioning—Glasgow Coma Scale, level of orientation, safety
Orthopedic complications—type of fractures, amputations
Other organ system complications—liver, lungs
Prognosis
Anticipated long-term disability
Rehabilitation potential
On-the-job injury

FORM A1-1

GENERIC SCREENING CRITERIA FOR OPENING CASE MANAGEMENT CASES

Telephonic Versus On-Site

PATIENT NAME:______________________________

SOCIAL SECURITY NUMBER:______________________

PAYER:____________________________________

1. Catastrophic or chronic diagnosis amenable to case management intervention. Y N

   Comments:____

   ____

2. Prolonged hospital stay expected or has already occurred, frequent hospitalizations/frequent ER visits. Y N

   Comments:____

   ____

3. Questionable adequacy of the facility or provider based on patient's condition/needs. Y N

   Comments:____

   ____

4. Treatment/discharge plans in need of clarification/modification. Y N

   Comments:____

   ____

5. Potential opportunity for rate negotiations with providers/vendors. Y N

   Comments:____

   ____

6. Potential opportunity for safely reducing level of care. Y N

   Comments:____

   ____

Two or more positive responses are strong indicators of the appropriateness of full case management services and an on-site visit.

FORM A1-2

CRITERIA FOR DETERMINING ORDER OF PRECEDENCE FOR CASE MANAGEMENT SERVICES

PATIENT NAME:______________________________

SOCIAL SECURITY NUMBER:______________________

PAYER:____________________________________

	RANK WEAK–STRONG	WEIGHT MULTIPLE BY RANK	SCORE
1. Possible quality issues	1 2 3 4 5	3	______
2. Potential for high dollar cost savings	1 2 3 4 5	3	______

Comments:____

____

3. Urgency to facilitate discharge/treatment plan	1 2 3 4 5	1	______

Comments:____

____

4. Problems with coordination of care	1 2 3 4 5	3	______

Comments:____

____

5. Number of complicating factors	1 2 3 4 5	1	______

Comments:____

____

6. Acuity level of patient	1 2 3 4 5	1	______

Total score = ________

Immediate need for case management intervention—40-50 total score

Medium need for case management intervention—26-39 total score

Lower need for case management intervention (further research)—10-25 total score

APPENDIX 2

DEVELOPING AND USING LETTERS AND FORMS FOR CASEWORK

CONTENTS

A Examples of Case Management Forms

1. ***Case Management Request Form*** *(Form A2-1)*
   A useful tool for both referral sources and case managers. The request form outlines the pertinent information needed to perform a case management screening and also outlines what the referral source can expect from the case manager. As the case is worked, the issues listed on these forms serve as a method of measuring case progress and ensuring that all of the referral questions and concerns are being adequately addressed.

2. ***Client/Family Interview Form*** *(Form A2-2)*
   Provides a structured format for the case manager during the initial assessment phase of the case management process. The interview form outlines specific information that the case manager must obtain to begin to effectively work a case.

3. ***Health Care Provider Interview Form*** *(Form A2-3)*
   Outlines information to be obtained from physicians or other health care providers concurrently working with a patient. The health care provider interview form is a useful tool to complete at team conferences or in one-on-one meetings with physicians.

4. ***Cost Savings Measurement Form for Case Management Cases*** *(Form A2-4)*
   Provides case managers with a tool to capture and calculate cost savings.

5. ***Patient Care Assessment Form*** *(Form A2-5)*
   Gives the case manager a format to examine the functional abilities of the patient to perform activities of daily living, the barriers to a return to independence, and specific skilled care requirements. The form outlines medical treatments required and can be used to match an individual patient's skilled care needs with a specific placement, that is, skilled home care or a skilled nursing facility.

6. ***Health Care Facility/Agency Questionnaire*** *(Form A2-6)*
   Outlines the staffing, services, and pricing for health care facilities or agencies. It is a useful tool for evaluating a specific facility/agency for either individual placement or for participation in a preferred provider agreement.

7. ***Medical Case Management Authorization to Secure and Release Information*** *(Form A2-7)*
   This form is used to cover both release of information to others and obtaining information from others. Because laws governing confidentiality of information and privacy vary from jurisdiction to jurisdiction, each firm needs to develop forms that comply with appropriate legislation.

8 ***Contact Sheet*** *(Form A2-8)*
Documents all interventions made by the case manager and is used for billing purposes to determine the time spent on the case.

B Report Writing Formats

1 ***Initial Case Management Report*** *(Form A2-9)*
The first report on case management assessments, interventions, and recommendations forwarded to the client. Case managers should use the following guidelines unless they are specifically modified by the customer. The initial evaluation should include the following:

- *Reason for referral:* Identifies who referred the case, why the case was referred, and the primary diagnosis
- *Health care providers:* Names, addresses, and phone numbers of all pertinent health care providers
- *History of current illness:* A chronologic review of medical history, discussion of current treatment plan, and potential or actual complications of the disease or treatment plan
- *Medical systems affected by current illness:* System by system review of any system that is affected by the patient's status
- *Psychosocial implications:* A review of support systems, financial issues, community resources, compliance issues, and coping strategies
- *Case management interventions:* Qualitative discussion of on-site visits, review of any and all coordination performed by the case manager, and overview of planned future interventions
- *Cost analysis:* Discussion of both hard and soft dollar cost savings
- *Goals:* Both long-term and short-term goals should be identified
- *Summary and recommendations:* Summary of all pertinent aspects of the case along with recommendations for specific client and case management activities. Ongoing case management authorization should be addressed here.

2 ***Initial Case Management Report: Psychiatric and Chemical Dependency*** *(Form A2-10)*

3 ***Case Management Status Update/Progress Report*** *(Form A2-11)*
The frequency and contact of progress reports should be cleared with the client. The status update/progress reports should include the following:

- *Review of current status:* Brief update on medical condition, discussion of any changes in patient status, or changes in the treatment plan since last reporting date
- *Case management interventions:* Discussion of all interventions made since last reporting, including any cost-savings updates; also should include rationale for ongoing case management
- *Recommendations:* Summary of future activities and ongoing authorization for case management intervention

4 ***Case Management Final Report*** *(Form A2-12)*
Should be written in a timely manner while determining to close a case and should include the following:

- *Reason for original referral:* Identifies who referred the case, why the case was referred, and the primary diagnosis
- *Summary of case status:* Brief update on medical condition, discussion of any changes in patient status, or changes in the treatment plan since last reporting date
- *Case management interventions:* Discussion of interventions and rationale for closing case
- *Cost savings:* Brief overview of all hard and soft dollar cost savings, with in-depth discussion of ways that case manager was able to affect the patient's quality of life

- *Recommendations and summary:* Review of rationale for closure of case and specific recommendations for customer to watch for future claims activity

C Examples of Form Letters

1 *Letter Confirming Medical Appointment* *(Box A2-1)*
Confirms an appointment with the physician made for the client by the case manager; primarily used in vocational rehabilitation for independent medical examinations.

2 *Job Offer Confirmation Letter* *(Box A2-2)*
Sent to the client (usually in a workers' compensation case) to confirm an employment offer; it is helpful if it is sent by certified mail so that receipt can be verified.

3 *Request for Benefits Exception* *(Box A2-3)*
Sent by case manager to payer to obtain written verification for allocation of extracontractual benefits for the client.

4 *Introduction to Case Management Letter to Client/Family* *(Box A2-4)*
The first written contact that the client has from the case manager. The goal is to introduce both the case manager and the case management role to the client and family.

5 *Letter to Referral Source Acknowledging Receipt of Referral* *(Box A2-5)*
Sent by the case manager to the referral source to verify that the referral has been received and that case management is appropriate. It also confirms in writing the hours that are allowed for work on the case.

6 *Letter to Referral Source Recommending That Client Be Placed on "Watch Status"* *(Box A2-6)*
Outlines the reasons why a case is not appropriate for case management at this time and specific activities that the referral source should watch for in the future.

7 *Letter to Referral Source Recommending That Client Not Be Referred to Case Management* *(Box A2-7)*
Updates referral source on reasons why case management is not appropriate for a specific patient.

8 *Letter of Introduction to Physician* *(Box A2-8)*
Introduces the case manager to the physician, verifies proper release of information from the client, and begins the process of collaboratively working on the case.

FORM A2-1

CASE MANAGEMENT REQUEST FORM

PATIENT NAME: ______________________________

ADDRESS: ______________________________

____

____

DATE OF BIRTH: ______________________________

PHONE: (W): ______________________________

(H): ______________________________

SOCIAL SECURITY NUMBER: ______________________________

INSURED NAME: ______________________________

INSURED SOCIAL SECURITY NUMBER: ______________________________

DATE OF REFERRAL: ______________________________

PAYER: ______________________________

CONTACT: ______________________________

DATE OF ILLNESS: ______________________________

PRIMARY DIAGNOSIS: ______________________________

PRIMARY CARE PHYSICIAN: ______________________________

____

SPECIALIST PHYSICIAN: ______________________________

____

PHONE: ______________________________

Insurance eligibility and benefit coverage limits: ______________________________

____

____

Other providers: ______________________________

____

____

____

Reason for referral: ______________________________

____

____

Referral source expectations: ______________________________

____

____

____

____

Case management hours authorized: ______________________________

Timeline for next requested update: ______________________________

FORM A2-2

CLIENT/FAMILY INTERVIEW FORM

PATIENT NAME: ______________________________

DATE OF INTERVIEW: ______________________________

CASE MANAGER: ______________________________

1. Brief medical history ____

____

____

____

____

2. Patient/family perception of diagnosis/prognosis ______________________________

____

____

____

____

3. Patient/family assessment of treatment plan ______________________________

____

____

____

____

4. Patient/family goals for treatment plan and review of potential barriers ______________

____

____

____

____

5. Psychosocial factors ____

____

____

____

____

FORM A2-3

HEALTH CARE PROVIDER INTERVIEW FORM

DATE OF INTERVIEW: ____________________ PATIENT NAME: ____________________

PROVIDER NAME: ____________________ CASE MANAGER: ____________________

1. Diagnosis—Primary: ____________________

   Secondary: ____________________
2. Brief history of current illness (include treatment, medications, and possible complications)

   Symptoms: ____________________

   Treatment: ____________________

   Medications: ____________________
3. Systems review:
   a. Neurologic/psychiatric system
   b. Gastrointestinal system
   c. Visual and auditory system
   d. Pulmonary system
   e. Integumentary system
   f. Genitourinary system
   g. Musculoskeletal system
   h. Endocrine system
4. Psychosocial status
5. Prognosis
6. Projected discharge date
7. Discharge needs (care, equipment, and treatment)
8. Patient compliance (cooperation), attitude toward illness
9. Education
10. Other

FORM A2-4

COST SAVINGS MEASUREMENT FORM FOR CASE MANAGEMENT CASES

1. A. Reduction in length of stay in specialized unit (________________) by________________

____

Expected stay of ________ days × $________ / day = $________________

Actual care of ________ days × $________ / day = $________________

Gross savings = $________________

B. Reduction in length of stay in acute care unit by ________________________________

____

____

Expected stay of ________ days × $________ / day = $________________

Gross savings = $________________

C. Reduction in length of stay in rehabilitation/long-term care unit (________________) by

____

____

Expected stay of ________ days × $________ / day = $________________

Actual care of ________ days × $________ / day = $________________

Gross savings = $________________

2. Avoidance of admission or readmission to ________________ unit by________________

____

Potential of________ days × $________ / day = $________________

Actual care of ________ days × $________ / day = $________________

Gross savings = $________________

3. Implementation of home health care in lieu of hospitalization by________________

____

If hospitalized for________ days × $________ / day = $________________

Home care for ________ days × $________ / day = $________________

Gross savings = $________________

Continued

FORM A2-4

COST SAVINGS MEASUREMENT FORM FOR CASE MANAGEMENT CASES—cont'd

4. Decrease in level of home health care by ____________________

____

Previously __________ for __________/hours × = $ __________

Actually __________ for __________/hours × = $ __________

Gross savings = $ __________/day

= $ __________/week

5. Decrease in hours/day or days/week of home health care by ____________________

____

Previously __________ hours/day × $__________ / day = $ __________/day

OR __________ hours/day × $__________ / day = $ __________/week

Actually __________ hours/day × $__________ / day = $ __________/day

OR __________ hours/day × $__________ / day = $ __________/week

Gross savings = $ __________/day

= $ __________/week

6. Decrease in cost of equipment and supplies by ____________________

____

Previous cost $____________________

Actual cost $____________________

Gross savings $ ____________________

7. Decrease in therapy (__________) by ____________________

____

Previously ______ sessions/week × $ ______/session = $__________

Actually ______ sessions/week × $ ______/session = $__________

Gross savings = $ __________/week

8. Other cost savings: ____________________

____

____

____

FORM A2-4

COST SAVINGS MEASUREMENT FORM FOR CASE MANAGEMENT CASES—cont'd

Gross savings: 1.A. $____________________

1.B. $____________________

1.C. $____________________

2. $____________________

3. $____________________

4. $____________________

5. $____________________

6. $____________________

7. $____________________

8. $____________________

Total gross savings: $____________________

Cost of case management: $____________________

Net savings: $____________________ per month/year

Return on investment: $____________________ per $1.00

FORM A2-5

PATIENT CARE ASSESSMENT FORM

A. Demographics

PATIENT NAME: ____________________ AGE: ____________________

COMPANY FILE NUMBER: ____________________ SEX: ____________________

SOCIAL SECURITY NUMBER: ____________________ MARITAL STATUS: ____________________

PRIMARY DIAGNOSIS: ____________________ HEIGHT: ____________________

SECONDARY DIAGNOSIS: ____________________ WEIGHT: ____________________

____________________ DATE OF BIRTH: ____________________

EMPLOYER/PLAN SPONSOR: ____________________ ATTENDING PHYSICIAN: ____________________

B. General care requirements

1. Level of care recommended: ____________________
2. Number of hours of care recommended: ____________________
3. Length of time care projected: ____________________

C. Specific patient needs

1. *Eating* Diet ________ Supervised/minimal assistance ________
   Independent ________ Set up tray ________ Must be fed ________
2. *Toileting* Independent ________ Some assistance ________ Total assistance ________
   Occasional accident ________ Nocturnal incontinence ________
   Frequent bladder incontinence ________ Bowel incontinence ________
3. *Bathing* Independent ________ Needs supervision only ________
   Must be bathed ________ Assistance in/out of tub ________
4. *Dressing and grooming* Independent ________
   Needs assistance ________ Supervision only ________
5. *Transferring and positioning*
   Independent ________ Independent with device ________
   Aid of one person ________ Aid of two people ________
   Unable ________

FORM A2-5

PATIENT CARE ASSESSMENT FORM—cont'd

C. Specific patient needs—cont'd

6. *Need for restraint* Frequently ____________ Occasionally ____________

   Always ____________ Never ____________

7. *Wheeling* Independent _______ Minimal assistance _______ Total assistance _______

8. *Ambulation* Independent ____________ Independent with device ____________

   Aid of one person ___________ Aid of two persons ___________ Unable ___________

9. *Wandering* Wanders ____________ Does not wander ____________

10. *Vision* Normal ___________ Partial impairment ___________ Unable ___________

11. *Hearing* Normal ___________ Partial impairment ___________ Unable ___________

12. *Communication*

    Normal speech ____________ Speech impairment ____________

    Language barrier ____________ Inappropriate content ____________

    Makes needs known with difficulty ____________ Unable to speak ____________

13. *Behavior—disoriented*

    Never ____________ Occasionally ____________ Frequently ____________

    Severely/always ____________

14. *Behavior—impaired judgment*

    Never ____________ Occasionally ____________ Frequently ____________

    Severely/always ____________

15. *Pain management*

    None required ____________ Some management ____________

    Moderate management ____________ Difficult to manage ____________

16. *Perceptual motor function*

    Normal ____________ Partial impairment ____________ Unable ____________

17. *Cooperation with treatment regimen*

    Never ____________ Occasionally ____________ Frequently ____________

    Always ____________

18. *Family/social support* None ____________ Occasionally ____________

    Frequently ____________ Always ____________

Continued

FORM A2-5
PATIENT CARE ASSESSMENT FORM—cont'd

D. Medications

NAME	FREQUENCY	DOSE

E. Treatments/therapies — FREQUENCY

1. Inhalation treatment ______________
2. Oxygen ______________
3. Suctioning ______________
4. Vital signs ______________
5. Indwelling catheter ______________
6. Catheter/tube irrigation ______________
7. IV therapy ______________
8. Ostomy care ______________
9. Tube feeding ______________
10. Decubiti care ______________
11. Minor skin care/dressing ______________
12. Intake and output ______________
13. Physical therapy ______________
14. Occupational therapy ______________
15. Speech therapy ______________
16. Social work services ______________
17. Mental health counseling ______________
18. Chemical dependency counseling ______________
19. Vocational counseling ______________
20. Physiatry services ______________

FORM A2-5

PATIENT CARE ASSESSMENT FORM—cont'd

E. Treatments/therapies—cont'd

	FREQUENCY
21. Recreational therapy	______________
22. Behavior modification services	______________
23. Dietary counseling	______________
24. Cognitive reeducation	______________
25. Family support groups	______________

F. Other comments

1. Other nursing care needs:
2. Benefit plan considerations:
3. Brief summary of case:

______________________________ ______________

REPRESENTATIVE SIGNATURE DATE

FORM A2-6

HEALTH CARE FACILITY/AGENCY QUESTIONNAIRE

AGENCY NAME: ______________________

____

ADDRESS: ______________________

____

____

TELEPHONE NUMBER: ______________________

FAX NUMBER: ______________________

CONTACT PERSON: ______________________

____

I. Administration/facility

A. Current licensure: ______________________
(e.g., SNF, RTF)

B. Specialty certification: ______________________
(e.g., CARF, JCAHO)

C. Target patient population: ______________________

D. Visiting hours: ______________________

E. Hallways, rooms, and restrooms handicapped accessible: ______________________

F. Describe routine daily activities: ______________________

____

II. Staffing

A. Nursing to resident ratio per shift

______________ DAY

______________ EVENING

______________ NIGHT

B. Number of RNs on each shift

______________ DAY

______________ EVENING

______________ NIGHT

C. Number of LPNs on each shift

______________ DAY

______________ EVENING

______________ NIGHT

FORM A2-6

HEALTH CARE FACILITY/AGENCY QUESTIONNAIRE—cont'd

II. Staffing—cont'd

D. Number of other professional staff regularly available on each shift

_______________ DAY

_______________ EVENING

_______________ NIGHT

E. Types of other professional staff routinely available: _______________

III. Services

Describe the following services provided in your facility:

SERVICE	YES	NO	AVAILABLE ON CALL	MAY BE ARRANGED
1. Inhalation	______	______	______	______
2. Oxygen	______	______	______	______
3. Suctioning	______	______	______	______
4. Vital signs	______	______	______	______
5. Indwelling catheter	______	______	______	______
6. Catheter/tube irrigation	______	______	______	______
7. IV therapy	______	______	______	______
8. Ostomy care	______	______	______	______
9. Tube feeding	______	______	______	______
10. Decubiti care	______	______	______	______
11. Minor skin care/dressing	______	______	______	______
12. Intake and output	______	______	______	______
13. Physical therapy	______	______	______	______
14. Occupational therapy	______	______	______	______
15. Speech therapy	______	______	______	______
16. Social work services	______	______	______	______
17. Mental health counseling	______	______	______	______
18. Chemical dependency counseling	______	______	______	______
19. Vocational counseling	______	______	______	______

Continued

FORM A2-6

HEALTH CARE FACILITY/AGENCY QUESTIONNAIRE—cont'd

III. Services—cont'd

Service	Yes	No	Available On Call	May Be Arranged
20. Physiatry services	______	______	______	______
21. Recreational therapy	______	______	______	______
22. Behavior modification services	______	______	______	______
23. Dietary counseling	______	______	______	______
24. Cognitive reeducation	______	______	______	______
25. Family support groups	______	______	______	______

IV. Other services

Service	Yes	No	Available On Call	May Be Arranged
1. Physician	______	______	______	______
2. Dentist	______	______	______	______
3. Spiritual/religious services	______	______	______	______
4. Barber/beautician services	______	______	______	______
5. Transportation services	______	______	______	______

V. Patient population

A. Diagnosis(es) appropriate for facility: ______________________________

____

B. Age mix for facility: ______________________________

Range: ______________________________

Means: ______________________________

C. Medicaid/Medicare/private patient mix: ______________________________

D. Resident's role in forming policies: ______________________________

VI. Costs

A. State the basic rate and the services covered by this basic rate: ______________________________

____

FORM A2-6

HEALTH CARE FACILITY/AGENCY QUESTIONNAIRE—cont'd

VI. Costs—cont'd

B. Describe the services/treatments that are extra and the associated costs:

EXTRA SERVICES/TREATMENT	ASSOCIATED COSTS

VII. Interface with case manager

A. Frequency of multidisciplinary team meetings:____________________

____

B. Availability of case manager to attend multidisciplinary team meetings:____________________

____

C. Willingness to share progress notes and reports with case manager: ____________________

____

VIII. Summary and Comments____________________

____

____

____________________ ____________________

REPRESENTATIVE SIGNATURE DATE

FORM A2-7

MEDICAL CASE MANAGEMENT
AUTHORIZATION TO SECURE AND RELEASE INFORMATION

PATIENT: ______________________________ **SOCIAL SECURITY NUMBER:** ____________________

I authorize the release to and use by ______________________, or any designee acting on the company's behalf, of any personal, medical, and employment-related information for myself or on behalf of my eligible dependents.

This information may be released by my attending physician or other medical professionals who have treated me. This information specifically may include details relating to alcohol or drug treatment, mental health treatment, communicable diseases such as hepatitis or HIV, or any other medical condition or treatment.

I fully understand that the intent of this authorization to secure information is solely for the purpose of case management and/or rehabilitation plan development on behalf of ______________________ (client or their contractually specific designee). I understand that ______________________ will release only information necessary to arrange medical and/or social services.

This authorization will remain in effect for one year from the date noted below while I am receiving case management services. I understand that I may withdraw this consent at any time except to the extent that action has already been taken.

I have a right to receive a copy of this authorization if I so request. A photostat of this authorization shall be as valid as the original.

______________________________ ____________________

PATIENT/PATIENT REPRESENTATIVE **DATE**

FORM A2-8

CONTACT SHEET

PATIENT: ______________________ FILE NUMBER: ______________________

TYPE OF SERVICE: ______________________

DATE	ACTIVITY	TIME	EXPENSES	NOTES

Total hours and expenses:

______________________ ______________

REPRESENTATIVE DATE

FORM A2-9

INITIAL CASE MANAGEMENT REPORT

TO: ______________________________

____

ATTN: ______________________________

____

FROM: ______________________________

____

____

DATE OF REPORT: ______________________________

PATIENT NAME: ______________________________

SOCIAL SECURITY NUMBER: ______________________________

Reason for referral ______________________________

____

Health care providers ______________________________

____

History of current illness ______________________________

____

Medical systems affected by current illness ______________________________

____

Psychosocial implications ______________________________

____

Case management interventions ______________________________

____

Cost analysis ______________________________

____

Goals ______________________________

____

Summary and recommendations ______________________________

____

FORM A2-10

INITIAL CASE MANAGEMENT REPORT: PSYCHIATRIC AND CHEMICAL DEPENDENCY

TO: ______________________________

____

ATTN: ______________________________

____

FROM: ______________________________

____

____

DATE OF REPORT: ______________________________

PATIENT NAME: ______________________________

SOCIAL SECURITY NUMBER: ______________________________

Reason for referral ______________________________

____

Health care providers ______________________________

History of current illness ______________________________

Axis 1 (Clinical syndromes and V codes) ______________________________

Axis 2 (Developmental disorders and personality disorders) ______________________________

Axis 3 (Physical disorders and conditions) ______________________________

Axis 4 (Severity of psychosocial stressors) ______________________________

Axis 5 (Global assessment of functioning) ______________________________

Psychosocial implications ______________________________

____

Case management interventions ______________________________

____

Cost analysis ______________________________

____

Goals ______________________________

____

Summary and recommendations ______________________________

____

FORM A2-11

CASE MANAGEMENT STATUS UPDATE/PROGRESS REPORT

TO: ____________________

____

ATTN: ____________________

____

FROM: ____________________

____

____

DATE OF REPORT: ____________________

PATIENT NAME: ____________________

SOCIAL SECURITY NUMBER: ____________________

Review of current status ____________________

____

____

Case management interventions ____________________

____

____

Recommendations ____________________

____

____

FORM A2-12

CASE MANAGEMENT FINAL REPORT

TO: ______________________________ DATE OF REPORT: ______________________________

______________________________ PATIENT NAME: ______________________________

ATTN: ______________________________ SOCIAL SECURITY NUMBER: ______________________________

____

FROM: ______________________________

____

____

Reason for original referral ______________________________

____

____

Summary of case status ______________________________

____

____

Case management interventions ______________________________

____

____

Cost savings ______________________________

____

____

Recommendations and summary ______________________________

____

____

BOX A2-1

LETTER CONFIRMING MEDICAL APPOINTMENT

[*Date*]

[*Client's name and address*]
Re: [*Insert*]
Dear [*Client's name*]:

This letter is to confirm that you have an appointment for an independent medical examination with Dr. [*name*] at [*location and address*] on [*date and time*].

Dr. [*name*] requires that you give him/her 24 hours advance notice if you need to reschedule this appointment. Please phone his/her office at [*phone number*] to reschedule. If you have to reschedule, would you also phone me at [*phone number*]? Enclosed is a map to Dr. [*name*]'s office.

Sincerely,

[*Case manager's name*]
Case Manager I
cc: [*Name and title*]
Enclosure(s): [*Description*]

BOX A2-2

JOB OFFER CONFIRMATION LETTER

[*Date*]

[*Client's name and address*]
Re: [*Insert*]
Dear [*Client's name*]:

This letter is to confirm that you have been offered the position of [*job title*] with [*employer's name*], which is scheduled to begin on [*date and time*] at [*location*]. Please let us know whether you will accept this job offer by [*date*]. If we do not hear from you by this date, we will assume that you have chosen to refuse this offer of employment. If you have any question about this or any issues to discuss, please phone me at [*phone number*].

Good luck with your new job.

Sincerely,

[*Case manager's name*]
Case Manager I
cc: [*Name and title*]
Enclosure(s): [*Description*]

BOX A2-3

REQUEST FOR BENEFITS EXCEPTION

[*Date*]

[*Payer's name and address*]
Re: [*Client's name*]
Dear [*Payer's name*]:

This letter is written to obtain acknowledgement of the receipt of and agreement with the recommendations for a benefits exception as presented in the enclosed report. Please note your receipt of the recommendations and approval of activity or note changes in plan or benefit below.

Thank you for taking the time to consider this request. Please feel free to call me with any questions or concerns on this matter.

Sincerely,

[*Case manager's name*]
Case Manager I

Please return a copy of this letter, with your signature, indicating your agreement with the request for a benefits exception.

____
Signature
cc: [*Name and title*]
Enclosure(s): [*Description*]

BOX A2-4

INTRODUCTION TO CASE MANAGEMENT LETTER TO CLIENT/FAMILY

[*Date*]

[*Client's name and address*]
Dear [*Client's name*]:

This letter is written to introduce myself to you and your family. I am a Registered Nurse and I work for [*company name*]. I have been requested by your health benefits carrier, [*payer name*], to assist you with health care benefits and coordination at this time. My role as a case manager is to work collaboratively with you to obtain the best and most appropriate health care services under your benefits plan. I look forward to talking with you. If you have any questions about this or any issues to discuss, please phone me at [*phone number*].

Sincerely,

[*Case manager's name*]
Case Manager I
Enclosure(s): [*Case management description*]

BOX A2-5

LETTER TO REFERRAL SOURCE ACKNOWLEDGING RECEIPT OF REFERRAL

[*Date*]

[*Payer's name and address*]
Re: [*Client's name*]
Dear [*Payer's name*]:

Thank you for this referral to Case Management services. [*Client's name*] is appropriate for full case management services based on [*outline specific rationale, including diagnosis and care needs*]. I would recommend [*specify hours*] of case management services to perform the initial assessment and evaluation for this client.

Please feel free to call me with any questions or concerns on this matter.

Sincerely,

[*Case manager's name*]
Case Manager I
Please return a copy of this letter, with your signature, indicating your agreement with the recommended number of hours of case management services.

____
Signature
cc: [*Name and title*]
Enclosure(s): [*Description*]

BOX A2-6

LETTER TO REFERRAL SOURCE RECOMMENDING THAT CLIENT BE PLACED ON "WATCH STATUS"

[*Date*]

[*Payer's name and address*]
Re: [*Client's name*]
Dear [*Payer's name*]:

Thank you for this referral to Case Management services. [*Client's name*] is not appropriate for full case management services at this time based on [*outline specific rationale*]. I would recommend that you continue to monitor [*client's name*] for future claims or any acute inpatient admissions. In the event that you become aware of a change in status, please contact me, and I will reevaluate the situation for appropriate case management services.

Please feel free to call me with any questions or concerns on this matter.
Sincerely,

[*Case manager's name*]
Case Manager I
cc: [*Name and title*]
Enclosure(s): [*Description*]

BOX A2-7

LETTER TO REFERRAL SOURCE RECOMMENDING THAT CLIENT NOT BE REFERRED TO CASE MANAGEMENT

[*Date*]

[*Payer's name and address*]
Re: [*Client's name*]
Dear [*Payer's name*]:

Thank you for this referral to Case Management services. [*Client's name*] is not appropriate for full case management services based on [*outline specific rationale*]. In order to assist you in identifying the most appropriate patients for case management, I would recommend that you not open [*client's name*] to case management at this time. In the event that [*client's name*] status changes, please contact me, and I will reevaluate the situation for appropriate case management services.

Please feel free to call me with any questions or concerns on this matter.
Sincerely,

[*Case manager's name*]
Case Manager I
cc: [*Name and title*]
Enclosure(s): [*Description*]

BOX A2-8

LETTER OF INTRODUCTION TO PHYSICIAN

[*Date*]

[*Physician's name and address*]
Re: [*Client's name*]
Dear [*Physician's name*]:

I am a Registered Nurse, employed by [*Company's name*]. I have been requested by [*company's name*] to work with you and [*client's name*] to provide health care coordination services. My role as a case manager is to work collaboratively with you and [*client's name*] to obtain the best and most appropriate health care services under your benefits plan. I look forward to talking with you.

I am enclosing a signed release of information from [*client's name*]. If you have any questions about this or any issues to discuss, please phone me at [*phone number*].

Sincerely,

[*Case manager's name*]
Case Manager I
Enclosure(s): [*Description*]

APPENDIX 3
VOCATIONAL REHABILITATION

CONTENTS

A The Vocational Rehabilitation/Evaluation Process

A step-by-step explanation of each stage of the vocational rehabilitation/evaluation process. Also includes a graphically illustrated example of how the process might progress from start to finish (Figure A3-1).

B Vocational History Form (Form A3-1)

A basic outline of the information that needs to be obtained during the initial interview with an injured worker or other vocational rehabilitation client. The information from this form is used for such purposes as transferrable skills analysis to determine employability.

C Job Analysis Form (Form A3-2)

This form contains a basic outline of information to be obtained during a job analysis (JA). JA involves the observation of a job or the interviewing of a worker to determine the components of the job and the requirements (physical abilities, skills, and background) to perform it. JAs can be obtained either in person or over the telephone.

D Labor Market Survey (LMS) Form (Form A3-3)

This form enables a vocational rehabilitation professional to obtain information about actual jobs from employers in the community. This information is used to supplement and verify information obtained during JAs.

E About the *Dictionary of Occupational Titles* (DOT)

This section quotes from the introduction to the DOT to give basic information on the development of the DOT and what is contained within it. Also includes information on how the DOT is used.

F About the *Classification of Jobs* (COJ), 1992 Revision

Basic information about another reference book that is often used by vocational rehabilitation counselors.

G Definitions from the DOT

This section also quotes directly from the DOT to explain concepts from the DOT that are commonly used in vocational rehabilitation and evaluation. These concepts include the following:

1. ***Specific Vocational Preparation (SVP)*** *(Box A3-1)*
2. ***General Educational Development (GED)*** *(Box A3-2)*
3. ***Physical Demands Strength Rating*** *(Box A3-3)*
4. ***Data, People, Things (DPT)*** *(Box A3-4)*
5. **Guide for Occupational Exploration *(GOE)*** *(Box A3-5)*

H Physical Capacities Evaluation (PCE) Form (Form A3-4)

An example of a form that is sent to physicians, panel examiners, physical therapists, and others to obtain information on the physical activities that an injured worker or other vocational client can reasonably be expected to perform without exacerbating his or her physical condition or experiencing undue discomfort.

THE VOCATIONAL REHABILITATION/EVALUATION PROCESS

The outline that follows details the individual steps within each stage of the vocational rehabilitation/evaluation process, as it is depicted in Figure A3-1.

Stage 1 Initial Vocational Assessment

- Client interview
  - Work history
  - Academic history
  - Skills inventory
  - Interest areas
- Medical information
  - Physical capacities evaluation (PCE)
  - Medical treatment plan
  - Restrictions
- Job analysis with current employer
  - Possible job modifications
  - Assessment of physical and other requirements
- Employability statement
  - Evaluation of client's current employability (regardless of number of actual job openings) in light of client's physical restrictions and vocational background

Stage 2 Other Job Possibilities Evaluated

- Transferrable skills analysis (manual or automated) to assess client's employability within physical restrictions and vocational background
- Job analysis (JA) of other jobs within client's physical and vocational capacities "as is"
- Job modifications and accommodations considered
- Rehabilitation engineering consultation possibly
- Labor market survey (LMS) conducted to assess job availability and requirements
- Work hardening to physically prepare client to return to work considered

Stage 3 Vocational Evaluation

- Paper and pencil tests (e.g., academic achievement)
- Work samples
- In-depth vocational history
- PCE and current medical history (including restrictions) obtained and reviewed
- Specific tests applicable to the client can be specified (e.g., neuropsychological tests for head-injured clients)
- Realistic job goal identified in light of physical capacities, academic abilities, and regulatory restrictions

Stage 4 Vocational Rehabilitation Plan

- Developed with all relevant medical, behavioral, and vocational information
- Considers physical capacities, work history, aptitudes, and direction provided from vocational evaluation
- Typically signed by client, attending physician, and case manager or vocational rehabilitation counselor
- Includes time frames, costs, and expected outcomes
- Client responsibilities, including consequences of noncompliance, and the role of the case manager or vocational rehabilitation counselor outlined

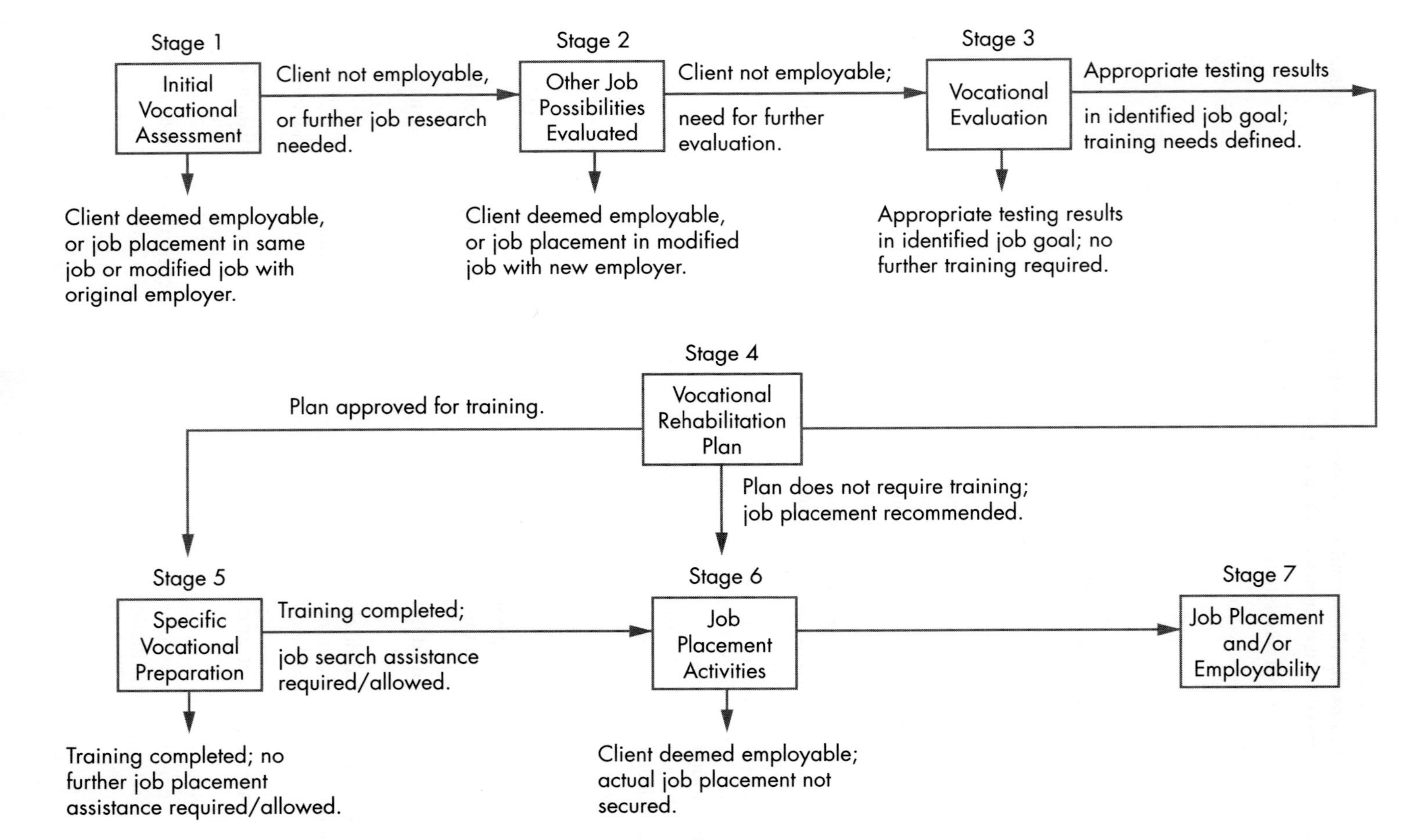

FIG. A3-1 Overview of vocational rehabilitation/evaluation process.

Stage 5 Specific Vocational Preparation

- Necessary vocational training identified, including availability, costs, location, transportation, accommodation issues, and other training arrangements
- Training costs and reimbursement coordinated with referral source
- Client progress monitored through training program, including contacts with instructors and receipt of grades
- Work hardening or sheltered workshop placement considered

Stage 6 Job Placement Activities

- Job placement specialist may be used to assist in job hunt
- Appropriate résumé developed
- Job interviewing skills counseling
- Job hunt process, procedure, and techniques
- Job tryout and/or on-the-job training (OJT)
- Government incentives explored for employers hiring people with disabilities
- Successful job placement is goal
- Follow-up with employer and client after job placement to assure appropriateness
- Some jurisdictions do not allow for job placement assistance, so client is referred to public sector agencies, employability established

Stage 7 Job Placement and/or Employability

- Job placement, with salary reported to referral source
- Physician and others informed of job placement
- Employability statement issued if job placement does not occur
- Some jurisdictions/coverage compensate for loss in wage earning capacity; others do not, so new salary may or may not be critical in job placement

FORM A3-1

VOCATIONAL HISTORY FORM

(To be included with Client/Family Interview Form, Form A2-2)

CLIENT NAME: ______________________ DATE: ______________________

SIGNATURE: ______________________ CLAIM NUMBER: ______________________

JOB AT TIME OF INJURY OR DISABILITY:

JOB TITLE: ______________________ DOT TITLE: ______________________

EMPLOYER: ______________________

DATES OF EMPLOYMENT: FROM __________ TO __________ TOTAL EXPERIENCE __________

NUMBER OF HOURS WORKED/WEEK: __________ SHIFT/HOURS: ______________________

Job duties ______________________

Tools/equipment used ______________________

Reason why job ended ______________________

Qualifications for job ______________________

PREVIOUS EMPLOYMENT

JOB TITLE: ______________________ DOT TITLE: ______________________

EMPLOYER: ______________________

DATES OF EMPLOYMENT: FROM __________ TO __________ TOTAL EXPERIENCE __________

NUMBER OF HOURS WORKED/WEEK: __________ SHIFT/HOURS: ______________________

Job duties ______________________

FORM A3-1

VOCATIONAL HISTORY FORM—cont'd

PREVIOUS EMPLOYMENT—cont'd

Tools/equipment used ______________________________

____

____

Reason why job ended ______________________________

Qualifications for job ______________________________

JOB TITLE: ______________ **DOT TITLE:** ______________

EMPLOYER: ______________________________

DATES OF EMPLOYMENT: FROM ________ **TO** ________ **TOTAL EXPERIENCE** ________

NUMBER OF HOURS WORKED/WEEK: ________ **SHIFT/HOURS:** ______________

Job duties ______________________________

____

____

____

____

Tools/equipment used ______________________________

____

____

Reason why job ended ______________________________

Qualifications for job ______________________________

JOB TITLE: ______________ **DOT TITLE:** ______________

EMPLOYER: ______________________________

DATES OF EMPLOYMENT: FROM ________ **TO** ________ **TOTAL EXPERIENCE** ________

NUMBER OF HOURS WORKED/WEEK: ________ **SHIFT/HOURS:** ______________

Job duties ______________________________

____

____

Continued

FORM A3-1

VOCATIONAL HISTORY FORM—cont'd

PREVIOUS EMPLOYMENT—cont'd

Tools/equipment used ______________________________

____

____

Reason why job ended ______________________________

Qualifications for job ______________________________

JOB TITLE: ______________ DOT TITLE: ______________

EMPLOYER: ______________________________

DATES OF EMPLOYMENT: FROM __________ TO __________ TOTAL EXPERIENCE __________

NUMBER OF HOURS WORKED/WEEK: __________ SHIFT/HOURS: ______________

Job duties ______________________________

____

____

____

____

Tools/equipment used ______________________________

____

____

Reason why job ended ______________________________

Qualifications for job ______________________________

EDUCATION/TRAINING

HIGHEST GRADE COMPLETED: __________ YEAR COMPLETED: __________

HIGH SCHOOL DIPLOMA: __________ GED: __________ YEAR: __________

COLLEGE NAME: ______________ MAJOR: ______________

DEGREE: ______________ YEARS ATTENDED: __________

VOCATIONAL SCHOOL: ______________ SUBJECT(S): ______________

COMPLETED: ______________ YEARS ATTENDED: __________

FORM A3-1

VOCATIONAL HISTORY FORM—cont'd

EDUCATION/TRAINING—cont'd

ON-THE-JOB TRAINING: ______________________ OCCUPATION: ______________________

COMPLETED: ____________ YEAR(S): __________

APPRENTICESHIP: ______________________ OCCUPATION: ______________________

COMPLETED: ____________ YEAR(S): __________

MILITARY: ______________________ JOB(S): ______________________

TYPE OF DISCHARGE: ______________________ SPECIAL TRAINING: ______________________

YEARS: __________

LICENSE/CERTIFICATES HELD: ______________________ YEAR(S): ______________________

DRIVER'S LICENSE: ______________________

HOBBIES, RECREATION, AND VOLUNTEER ACTIVITIES

____

____

____

GENERAL OCCUPATIONAL SKILLS

____

____

____

____

TEST SCORES

____

____

____

FORM A3-2

JOB ANALYSIS FORM

INJURED WORKER: ____________________ CLAIM NUMBER: ____________________

JOB TITLE: ____________________ DATE OF ANALYSIS: ____________________

EMPLOYER'S NAME: ____________________ ON-SITE OR PHONE ANALYSIS: ____________________

EMPLOYER'S ADDRESS: ____________________ JOB ANALYST: ____________________

____

EMPLOYER'S PHONE: ____________________

CONTACT PERSON: ____________________ TITLE: ____________________

DOT JOB TITLE: ____________________ DOT NUMBER: ____________________

PHYSICAL DEMANDS: ____________________ SVP: ____________________

GOE NUMBER: ____________________

Description of job ____

____

____

____

List of duties and responsibilities ____

____

____

____

HOURS WORKED PER DAY: ________ HOURS WORKED PER WEEK: ________ OVERTIME: ________

KEY

N	**Not present**	Activity or condition does not exist
R	**Rare**	Activity exists up to $1/8$ of time
O	**Occasionally**	Activity or condition exists from $1/8$ to $1/2$ of time
F	**Frequently**	Activity or condition exists from $1/2$ to $1/3$ of time
C	**Constantly**	Activity or condition exists $2/3$ or more of time

FORM A3-2

JOB ANALYSIS FORM—cont'd

ACTIVITY	HOURS AT A TIME	TOTAL HOURS	ADDITIONAL INFORMATION
Standing	______	______	Surface
Walking	______	______	Surface
			Distance
Sitting	______	______	Surface

Comments ____

____

LIFTING		WEIGHT IN POUNDS	N/A	RARE	OCCASIONALLY	FREQUENTLY	CONSTANTLY
Floor to waist	Normal	______	___	____	____	____	____
	Maximum	______	___	____	____	____	____
Waist to neck	Normal	______	___	____	____	____	____
	Maximum	______	___	____	____	____	____
Above neck	Normal	______	___	____	____	____	____
	Maximum	______	___	____	____	____	____

Comments ____

____

		WEIGHT IN POUNDS	N/A	RARE	OCCASIONALLY	FREQUENTLY	CONSTANTLY
Carrying	Normal	______	___	____	____	____	____
	Maximum	______	___	____	____	____	____
Pushing	Normal	______	___	____	____	____	____
	Maximum	______	___	____	____	____	____
Pulling	Normal	______	___	____	____	____	____
	Maximum	______	___	____	____	____	____

Comments ____

____

Continued

FORM A3-2

JOB ANALYSIS FORM—cont'd

Upper Extremity and Hand Function

	N/A	Rare	Occasionally	Frequently	Constantly
Grasping	______	______	______	______	______
Reaching	______	______	______	______	______
Above shoulder	______	______	______	______	______
Shoulder to waist	______	______	______	______	______
Below waist	______	______	______	______	______
Handling	______	______	______	______	______
Torquing	______	______	______	______	______
Fingering	______	______	______	______	______

Comments ____

____

Trunk Mobility

	N/A	Rare	Occasionally	Frequently	Constantly
Twisting	______	______	______	______	______
Bending	______	______	______	______	______
Crawling	______	______	______	______	______
Crouching	______	______	______	______	______

Comments ____

____

Lower Extremity

	N/A	Rare	Occasionally	Frequently	Constantly
Squatting	______	______	______	______	______
Kneeling	______	______	______	______	______
Climbing	______	______	______	______	______
Balancing	______	______	______	______	______
Operating foot controls	______	______	______	______	______

Comments ____

____

FORM A3-2

JOB ANALYSIS FORM—cont'd

Environmental conditions

INSIDE: ________%

OUTSIDE: ________%

TEMPERATURE EXTREMES: ________

FUMES: ________

DUST: ________

GASES: ________

ODORS: ________

MIST: ________

NOISE/VIBRATION: ________

Comments____

____

Sensory communication

HEARING: ________

SEEING: ________

SMELLING: ________

TALKING: ________

TASTING: ________

Comments____

____

Tools and equipment used__________________________________

____

Potential hazards____

____

Protective clothing or devices ______________________________

____

Potential for job modifications______________________________

____

________________________________ ____________

VOCATIONAL REHABILITATION COUNSELOR/CASE MANAGER **DATE**

Employer review:
I have read the above job analysis and believe it is an accurate representation of the job duties and physical requirements for this position.

________________________________ ____________

EMPLOYER SIGNATURE **DATE**

Continued

FORM A3-2

JOB ANALYSIS FORM—cont'd

Attending physician's response

Approved: Yes: _______ No: _______

If not approved, please indicate why ____

Would a job modification allow your patient to return to work? ____________ If so, please describe

____

____

When do you anticipate lifting the restrictions? ______________________________

Comments ____

____

______________________________ ______________

PHYSICIAN'S SIGNATURE DATE

FORM A3-3

LABOR MARKET SURVEY (LMS) FORM

JOB TITLE: ______________________ **DOT JOB TITLE:** ______________________

EMPLOYER: ______________________ **DOT NUMBER:** ______________________

EMPLOYER'S PHONE: ______________________ **SVP:** ______________________

PERSON CONTACTED: ______________________ **GOE CODE:** ______________________

TITLE: ______________________ **SURVEYOR:** ______________________

DATE OF CONTACT: ______________________

Essential tasks ______________________

____

Minimum qualifications ______________________

____

Physical demands ______________________

____

Other information ______________________

____

NUMBER OF POSITIONS THIS JOB TITLE: **DATE LAST HIRED:**

ANTICIPATED YEARLY HIRE: **CURRENT OPENINGS:**

HOURS PER DAY/WEEK: **WAGE/SALARY RANGE:**

FULL-TIME OR PART-TIME WORK AVAILABLE:

ABOUT THE DICTIONARY OF OCCUPATIONAL TITLES

The material that follows is quoted directly from the *Dictionary of Occupational Titles.* It provides a brief overview of the DOT's development, its contents, and its applications.

Introduction

The Dictionary of Occupational Titles *(DOT) was developed in response to the demand of an expanding public employment service for standardized occupational information to support job placement activities. The U.S. Employment Service recognized this need in the mid-1930's, soon after the passage of the Wagner-Peyser Act established a federal-state employment service system, and initiated an occupational research program, utilizing analysts located in numerous field offices throughout the country, to collect the information required. The use of this information has expanded from job matching applications to various uses for employment counseling, occupational and career guidance, and labor market information services.*

In order to properly match jobs and workers, the public employment service system requires that a uniform occupational language be used in all of its local job service offices. Highly trained occupational analysts must go out and collect reliable data which is provided to job interviewers so they may systematically compare and match the specifications of employer job openings with the qualifications of applicants who are seeking jobs through its facilities. The Occupational Analysis (OA) Program is currently supporting job analysis activity in the states of Michigan, Missouri, Massachusetts, and Utah, with North Carolina serving as the lead Field Center providing leadership and oversight.

Based on the data collected by occupational analysts, the first edition of the DOT was published in 1939. The first edition contained approximately 17,500 concise definitions presented alphabetically, by title, with a coding arrangement for occupational classification. Blocks of jobs were assigned 5 or 6-digit codes which placed them in one of 550 occupational groups and indicated whether the jobs were skilled, semi-skilled, or unskilled.

The second edition DOT, issued in March 1949, combined material in the first edition with several supplements issued throughout the World War II period. The second edition and its supplements reflected the impact of the war on jobs in the U.S. economy including new occupations in the plastics, paper and pulp, and radio manufacturing industries.

The third edition DOT, issued in 1965, eliminated the previous designation of a portion of the occupations as "skilled, semi-skilled, or unskilled" and substituted a classification system based on the nature of the work performed and the demands of such work activities upon the workers. These new indicators of work requirements included eight separate classification components: training time, aptitudes, interests, temperaments, physical demands, working conditions, work performed, and industry.

The fourth edition of the DOT published in 1977, contained over 2,100 new occupational definitions and several thousand other definitions were substantially modified or combined with related definitions. In order to document these changes, approximately 75,000 on-site job analysis studies were conducted from 1965 to the mid-1970's. These studies, supplemented by information obtained through extensive contacts with professional and trade associations, reflected the restructuring of the economy at that time.

Two supplements to the DOT have been released since the publication of the 1977 fourth edition DOT, one in 1982 and one in 1986. The 1982 supplement contained titles, codes, and definitions derived from Occupational Code Requests . . . submitted by DOT users to local Job service offices. The 1986 supplement continued this effort to publish new definitions as well as modify existing definitions consistent with new data collected. The 1986 supplement contained 840 occupational definitions; of these 761 were not defined in the fourth edition.

Changes in occupational content and job characteristics due to technological advancement continue to occur at a rapid pace. This rapid change to occupations coupled with user demand for the most current information possible has resulted in a revised approach to the publication of the DOT. The OA network has focused its efforts on the study of selected industries in order to document the jobs that have undergone the most significant occupational changes since the publication, in 1977, of the fourth edition DOT.

This effort of gathering data and writing/revising definitions in these selected industries, including "new" and revised definitions from the 1986 fourth edition supplement, has resulted in the publication of this revised fourth edition DOT.[131]

How to Use the DOT

- Look up the titles of all jobs and review other titles in the same section with the same specific vocational preparation (SVP). Some of these jobs may have different *Guide for Occupational Exploration* (GOE) designations.
- Review the Industry Index for possibilities.
- Use the date of the last update to compare work experience from previous years with the requirements of current jobs.

Companion Books to the DOT Published by the U.S. Government Printing Office (GPO)

These books are cross-referenced to the DOT through various codes:

- *Occupational Outlook Handbook*—revised biyearly
- *Selected Characteristics of Occupations Defined in the Revised DOT*—last edition 1993
- *Guide for Occupational Exploration*—currently out of print by the GPO but available in a new version through a private publisher, JIST[132]

Note: These books and the DOT are in the public domain "and may be reproduced fully or partially without the permission of the federal government. Source credit is requested but is not required."[133]

ABOUT THE *CLASSIFICATION OF JOBS* (COJ)—1992 REVISION

The *Classification of Jobs* is a reference book based on information developed by the U.S. Department of Labor, but it is published by a private company, Elliott & Fitzpatrick of Athens, Georgia.[134] This reference book consists of some information from the DOT that is organized in several different ways to facilitate transferrable skills analysis and to identify light and sedentary jobs that are related to a client's work history. Additional information relates to the General Aptitude Test Battery (GATB), a vocational test instrument developed and published by the U.S. Department of Labor. Some of the information contained in the COJ is also published in the *Selected Characteristics of Occupations Defined in the Revised DOT,* which is put out by the U.S. Department of Labor.

The following is a partial list of some of the information to be found in the COJ:

- Worker trait profiles of jobs and DOT and GOE codes
- 11 aptitude levels required by jobs; correspond to GATB scores
- Requirements for 20 types of physical demands
- 14 types of environmental conditions
- 11 temperaments

DEFINITIONS FROM THE DOT

The material in the five boxes that follow is quoted directly from the *Dictionary of Occupational Titles: fourth edition, revised 1991* to provide information on concepts that are commonly used or encountered in vocational rehabilitation and evaluation. The five concepts addressed here are as follows:

- Specific Vocational Preparation (SVP) (Box A3-1)
- General Educational Development (GED) (Box A3-2)
- Physical Demands Strength Rating (Box A3-3)
- Data, People, Things (Box A3-4)
- *Guide for Occupational Exploration* (GOE) (Box A3-5)

As with the information presented earlier in this Appendix, information from the DOT is in the public domain and may be reproduced fully or partially without the permission of the federal government. Source credit is requested but not required.

BOX A3-1

SPECIFIC VOCATIONAL PREPARATION (SVP)

Specific Vocational Preparation is defined as the amount of lapsed time required by a typical worker to learn the techniques, acquire the information, and develop the facility needed for average performance in a specific job-worker situation.

This training may be acquired in a school, work, military, institutional, or vocational environment. It does not include the orientation time required of a fully qualified worker to become accustomed to the special conditions of any new job. Specific vocational training includes vocational education, apprenticeship training, inplant training, on-the-job training, and essential experience in other jobs.

The following is an explanation of the various levels of specific vocational preparation:

LEVEL	TIME
1	Short demonstration only
2	Anything beyond short demonstration up to and including 1 month
3	Over 1 month up to and including 3 months
4	Over 3 months up to and including 6 months
5	Over 6 months up to and including 1 year
6	Over 1 year up to and including 2 years
7	Over 2 years up to and including 4 years
8	Over 4 years up to and including 10 years
9	Over 10 years

From *Dictionary of occupational titles: fourth edition, revised 1991*, Washington, DC, 1991, US Department of Labor, p 1009.

BOX A3-2

GENERAL EDUCATIONAL DEVELOPMENT (GED)

General Educational Development embraces those aspects of education (formal and informal) that are required of the worker for satisfactory job performance. This is education of a general nature that does not have a recognized, fairly specific occupational objective. Ordinarily, such education is obtained in elementary school, high school, or college. However, it may be obtained from experience and self-study.

The GED Scale is composed of three divisions: Reasoning Development, Mathematical Development, and Language Development. The descriptions of the various levels of language and mathematical development are based on the curricula taught in schools throughout the United States. An analysis of mathematics courses in school curricula reveals distinct levels of progression in the primary and secondary grades and in college. These levels of progression facilitated the selection and assignment of six levels of GED for the mathematical development scale.

However, though language courses follow a similar pattern of progression in primary and secondary school, particularly in learning and applying the principles of grammar, this pattern changes at the college level. The diversity of language courses offered at the college level precludes the establishment of distinct levels of language progression for these 4 years. Consequently, language development is limited to five defined levels of GED inasmuch as levels 5 and 6 share a common definition, even though they are distinct levels.

From *Dictionary of occupational titles: fourth edition, revised 1991*, Washington, DC, 1991, US Department of Labor, p 1009, 1012.

BOX A3-3

PHYSICAL DEMANDS STRENGTH RATING

The Physical Demands Strength Rating reflects the estimated overall strength requirement of the job expressed in terms of the letter corresponding to the particular strength rating. It represents the strength requirements that are considered to be important for average, successful work performance.

The strength rating is expressed by one of five terms: Sedentary, Light, Medium, Heavy, and Very Heavy. In order to determine the overall rating, an evaluation is made of the worker's involvement in the following activities:

a. Standing, Walking, Sitting

 Standing—Remaining on one's feet in an upright position at a workstation without moving about

 Walking—Moving about on foot

 Sitting—Remaining in a seated position

b. Lifting, Carrying, Pushing, Pulling

 Lifting—Raising or lowering an object from one level to another (including upward pulling)

 Carrying—Transporting an object, usually holding it in the hands or arms or on the shoulder

 Pushing—Exerting force on an object so that the object moves away from the force (includes slapping, striking, kicking, and treadle actions)

 Pulling—Exerting force on an object so that the object moves toward the force (includes jerking).

 Lifting, pushing, and pulling are evaluated in terms of both intensity and duration. Consideration is given to the weight handled, position of the worker's body, and the aid given by helpers or mechanical equipment. Carrying most often is evaluated in terms of duration, weight carried, and distance carried.

c. Controls

 Controls entail the use of one or both arms or hands (hand/arm) and/or one or both feet or legs (foot/leg) to move controls on machinery or equipment. Controls include but are not limited to buttons, knobs, pedals, levers, and cranks.

 Following are descriptions of the five terms in which the Strength Factor is expressed:

 S—Sedentary Work—Exerting up to 10 pounds of force occasionally (occasionally: activity or condition exists up to 1/3 of the time) and/or a negligible amount of force frequently (frequently: activity or condition exists from 1/3 to 2/3 of the time) to lift, carry, push, pull, or otherwise move objects, including the human body. Sedentary work involves sitting most of the time but may involve walking or standing for brief periods of time. Jobs are sedentary if walking and standing are required only occasionally and all other sedentary criteria are met.

BOX A3-3

PHYSICAL DEMANDS STRENGTH RATING—cont'd

L—Light Work—Exerting up to 20 pounds of force occasionally and/or up to 10 pounds of force frequently and/or a negligible amount of force constantly (constantly: activity or condition exists 2/3 or more of the time) to move objects. Physical demand requirements are in excess of those for Sedentary Work. Even though the weight lifted may be only a negligible amount, a job should be rated Light Work (1) when it requires walking or standing to a significant degree or (2) when it requires sitting most of the time but entails pushing and/or pulling of arm or leg controls and/or (3) when the job requires working at a production rate pace entailing the constant pushing and/or pulling of materials even though the weight of those materials is negligible. *Note:* The constant stress and strain of maintaining a production rate pace, especially in an industrial setting, can be and is physically demanding of a worker even though the amount of force exerted is negligible.

M—Medium Work—Exerting 20 to 50 pounds of force occasionally and/or 10 to 25 pounds of force frequently and/or greater than negligible up to 10 pounds of force constantly to move objects. Physical demand requirements are in excess of those for Light Work.

H—Heavy Work—Exerting 50 to 100 pounds of force occasionally and/or 25 to 50 pounds of force frequently and/or 10 to 20 pounds of force constantly to move objects. Physical demand requirements are in excess of those for Medium Work.

VH—Very Heavy Work—Exerting in excess of 100 pounds of force occasionally and/or in excess of 50 pounds of force frequently and/or in excess of 20 pounds of force constantly to move objects. Physical demand requirements are in excess of those for Heavy Work.

From *Dictionary of occupational titles: fourth edition, revised 1991*, Washington, DC, 1991, US Department of Labor, pp 1012-1013.

BOX A3-4

DATA, PEOPLE, THINGS (DPT)

Much of the information in [the DOT] is based on the premise that every job requires a worker to function, to some degree, in relation to Data, People, and Things. These relationships are identified and explained below. They appear in the form of three listings arranged in each instance from the relatively simple to the complex in such a manner that each successive relationship includes those that are simpler and excludes the more complex. (As each of the relationships to People represents a wide range of complexity, resulting in considerable overlap among occupations, their arrangement is somewhat arbitrary and can be considered a hierarchy only in the most general sense.) The identifications attached to these relationships are referred to as Worker Functions and provide standard terminology for use in summarizing how a worker functions on the job.

The fourth, fifth, and sixth digits of the occupational [DOT] code reflect relationships to Data, People, and Things, respectively. These digits express a job's relationship to Data, People, and Things by identifying the highest appropriate function in each listing shown in the following table:

DATA (4TH DIGIT)	PEOPLE (5TH DIGIT)	THINGS (6TH DIGIT)
0 Synthesizing	0 Mentoring	0 Setting Up
1 Coordinating	1 Negotiating	1 Precision Working
2 Analyzing	2 Instructing	2 Operating-Controlling
3 Compiling	3 Supervising	3 Driving-Operating
4 Computing	4 Diverting	4 Manipulating
5 Copying	5 Persuading	5 Tending
6 Comparing	6 Speaking-Signaling	6 Feeding-Offbearing
	7 Serving	7 Handling
	8 Taking Instructions-Helping	

From *Dictionary of occupational titles: fourth edition, revised 1991*, Washington, DC, 1991, US Department of Labor, p 1005.

BOX A3-5

GUIDE FOR OCCUPATIONAL EXPLORATION (GOE)

The *Guide for Occupational Exploration* was designed by the U.S. Employment Service to provide career counselors and other DOT users with additional information about the interests, aptitudes, entry level preparation, and other traits required for successful performance in various occupations. The GOE is also useful in self-assessment and counselor-assisted settings to help people understand themselves realistically in regard to their ability to meet job requirements. Descriptive information provided for each work group assists the individual in evaluating his or her own interests and relating them to pertinent fields of work.

The GOE code assigned to a [DOT] definition provides a link between the occupation defined [in the DOT] and the GOE arrangement of occupations with similar interests, aptitudes, adaptability requirements, and other descriptors.

The GOE coding structure classifies jobs at three levels of consideration. The first level divides occupations according to 12 interest areas corresponding to interest factors identified through research conducted by the former Division of Testing in the U.S. Employment Service. The interest factors, identified by a two-digit code, are defined in terms of broad interest requirements of occupations as well as vocational interests of individuals. The 12 interest areas are defined as follows:

01 Artistic
02 Scientific
03 Plants-Animals
04 Protective
05 Mechanical
06 Industrial
07 Business Detail
08 Selling
09 Accommodating
10 Humanitarian
11 Leading-Influencing
12 Physical Performing

The interest areas are then subdivided into work groups (the second set of two digits within the six-digit GOE code). Each work group contains occupations requiring similar worker traits and capabilities in related work settings. The GOE contains descriptive information for each work group and identifies each occupation in the group with a four-digit code and title. In many interest areas, occupations that require the most education, training, and experience are in the first group, whereas those requiring less formal education or experience are listed in the last group.

Work groups are then subdivided into subgroups (the third two-digit set in the GOE code) of occupations with even more homogeneous interests, aptitudes, and adaptability requirements. Each subgroup is identified by its unique six-digit code and title. Individual occupations are listed alphabetically within subgroups. Some subgroups contain occupations from more than one industry, listed within alphabetized industries.

Note: Although GOE codes are still used extensively for various purposes in vocational rehabilitation, the *Guide for Occupational Exploration* that was originally published through the U.S. Government Printing Office (GPO) is currently out of print. However, it has been replaced by the *Enhanced Guide for Occupational Exploration*, published by a private company.[135]

From *Dictionary of occupational titles: fourth edition, revised 1991*, Washington, DC, 1991, US Department of Labor, pp 1013-1014.

FORM A3-4

PHYSICAL CAPACITIES EVALUATION (PCE) FORM

CLIENT: ______________________ CLAIM NUMBER: ______________________

INSURER: ______________________ ATTENDING PHYSICIAN: ______________________

Instructions: Please rate this client's physical capacities in relationship to working a standard 8-hour day.

ACTIVITY	HOURS CAN PERFORM AT ONE TIME							TOTAL NUMBER OF HOURS PER DAY								
Sitting	1/4	1/2	1	2	3	4	5	0	1	2	3	4	5	6	7	8
Standing	1/4	1/2	1	2	3	4	5	0	1	2	3	4	5	6	7	8
Walking	1/4	1/2	1	2	3	4	5	0	1	2	3	4	5	6	7	8

ABLE TO PERFORM	CONTINUOUSLY	FREQUENTLY	OCCASIONALLY	RARELY	NEVER
Squatting	______	______	______	______	______
Twisting	______	______	______	______	______
Kneeling	______	______	______	______	______
Climbing	______	______	______	______	______
Bending/stooping	______	______	______	______	______
Reaching	______	______	______	______	______
Pushing/pulling	______	______	______	______	______
Fine Manipulation	______	______	______	______	______
Crawling	______	______	______	______	______

ABLE TO CARRY	CONTINUOUSLY	FREQUENTLY	OCCASIONALLY	RARELY	NEVER
0-10 lb	______	______	______	______	______
11-25 lb	______	______	______	______	______
26-35 lb	______	______	______	______	______
36-50 lb	______	______	______	______	______
51-75 lb	______	______	______	______	______
76-100 lb	______	______	______	______	______
Over 100 lb	______	______	______	______	______

FORM A3-4

PHYSICAL CAPACITIES EVALUATION (PCE) FORM—cont'd

ABLE TO LIFT	CONTINUOUSLY	FREQUENTLY	OCCASIONALLY	RARELY	NEVER
0-10 lb	______	______	______	______	______
11-25 lb	______	______	______	______	______
26-35 lb	______	______	______	______	______
36-50 lb	______	______	______	______	______
51-75 lb	______	______	______	______	______
76-100 lb	______	______	______	______	______
Over 100 lb	______	______	______	______	______

1. Client can use feet for repetitive movements such as operating foot controls:

   Right foot ____YES ____NO Left foot ____YES ____NO Both feet ____YES ____NO

2. Client can use hands for repetitive actions, such as:

	SIMPLE GRASPING	FIRM GRASPING	FINE MANIPULATION
Right hand	____YES ____NO	____YES ____NO	____YES ____NO
Left hand	____YES ____NO	____YES ____NO	____YES ____NO

3. Is this client able to work under the following environmental conditions?

Noise	____YES ____NO
Vibration	____YES ____NO
Unprotected heights	____YES ____NO
Cold	____YES ____NO
Heat	____YES ____NO
Fumes, gases, dust	____YES ____NO

Comments____

____

____

____

____

______________________________ ______________

PHYSICIAN'S SIGNATURE DATE

APPENDIX 4
CASE MANAGEMENT TEST

TEST QUESTIONS AND ANSWERS

1 **What is the basic purpose of case management?**
The basic purpose is coordination of quality health care services in a cost-effective manner. *Chapter 1.*

2 **What is a PPO?**
A PPO, a preferred provider organization, is a group of hospitals and physicians that contracts with employers, insurance carriers, third-party administrators, and other groups to supply comprehensive medical care services to subscribers and accept negotiated fee schedules as payment in full for services rendered. *Chapter 3.*

3 **What are the three major policies that exist under the accident and health side of the insurance industry, and which one is case management primarily involved with?**
Health/medical insurance, long-term disability, and accidental death and dismemberment policies. The type of accident and health coverage that is most likely to use case management services is health or medical insurance. *Chapter 5.*

4 **Name the four benefits allowed under workers' compensation.**
Medical benefits for coverage of health care services, cash benefits for nonfatal injury, cash benefits for fatal injuries, and rehabilitation benefits. *Chapter 5.*

5 **List six potential diagnoses that may be appropriate for case management screening.**
Traumatic brain injuries, severe burns, spinal cord injuries, AIDS , high-risk neonates, and organ transplants. *Chapter 7* and *Appendix 1.*

6 **What are the five steps in the case management process?**
Assessing, planning, coordinating, monitoring, and evaluation. *Chapter 1.*

7 **Briefly review what pertinent information the case manager should obtain from health care providers during the initial assessment.**
Diagnosis, history of the current illness or condition, review of systems, psychosocial status, prognosis, projected discharge date, discharge needs, and patient compliance. *Chapter 9.*

8 **Identify five types of negotiations that case managers may participate in or facilitate.**
Fee-for-service negotiations, per diem negotiations, case rate negotiations, purchase versus rental negotiations, and client placement. *Chapter 12.*

9 **What are the three different report formats that a case manager will typically complete while working a case?**
Opening, status updates, and closing reports. *Chapter 13.*

10 **Differentiate between work hardening and a transitional return to work.**
Work hardening programs are short-term programs during which a simulation of the physical requirements of the job is made to prepare the client for the rigors of the actual job. Transi-

tional return to work is part-time, light-duty work or gradually working into resuming full duties. *Chapter 16.*

11 **True of false: Substance abusers who are not current users and recovering alcoholics are not covered by the American with Disabilities Act (ADA).**
False. *Chapter 18.*

12 **True or false: Case managers are qualified to make denials of medical treatment based on medical necessity.**
False. *Chapters 6* and *19.*

Glossary

Accident and health insurance A line of insurance that pays medical and/or salary continuation benefits for conditions related to accidents and illness from events that are not insured by other lines, such as workers' compensation or liability insurance.

Accreditation Official certification by a recognized professional body that an organization or individual provider meets or exceeds a set of industry-derived standards.

Activities of daily living (ADLs) Tasks that are routinely performed by an individual on a daily basis, such as self-care, working, recreation, and caring for others.

Adjuster A person who handles insurance claims. May also be referred to as a claims manager, adjudicator, or claims examiner. Some adjusters pay medical-only claims; others handle property and indemnity.

Administrative services only (ASO) "An agency that delivers administrative services to an employer group. This type of arrangement usually requires the employer to be at risk for the cost of health care services provided."[136]

Alternate care A care setting that can serve as a substitute for an inpatient admission or nontraditional care. Some examples are outpatient surgery, home health care, acupuncture, and hospice.

Appeal This consists of a formal request for a review or a reconsideration of a determination. Appeals are usually made in writing and are in response to denials of medical services, vocational rehabilitation plans, or determinations of employability.

Attending physician/practitioner Although there may be more than one physician providing treatment to an individual, the attending physician is the one with the primary responsibility for care. For some managed care plans, midlevel practitioners (e.g., physician assistants and nurse practitioners) may serve as attending practitioners.

Authorization The approval granted by the third-party payer for such care as hospitalizations, durable medical equipment, or procedures. It also can refer to permission to proceed with case management services or recommendations.

Auto no-fault insurance In some states, automobile insurance is governed by no-fault laws, meaning that the carrier must cover the losses of the insured regardless of who is at fault.

Benefits The type, amount, or length of coverage provided by the insurance company.

Bill audit A review of provider bills for medical services, supplies, and equipment to identify errors or noncovered charges. In recent years, bill auditing has been extended to invoices of providers of case management and vocational rehabilitation services.

Board certified A physician who has met the requirements of a medical specialty board, including having passed the qualifying examination.

Board eligible A physician who meets the requirements of a medical specialty board to take the qualifying examination.

Capitation A type of payment for services in which a flat fee is charged per person regardless of the amount of individual consumption of services. The capitation usually covers a specific amount of time and can apply to medical services from a specific provider, utilization review services, case management services, and related services.

Carrier An insurance company or other entity, such as a self-insured employer, who indemnifies against loss.

Case management A collaborative process that assesses, plans, implements, coordinates, monitors, and evaluates options and services to meet an individual's health needs through communication and available resources to promote quality, cost-effective outcomes.

Chemical dependency services The diagnosis and treatment of drug, alcohol, and other chemical dependency.

Claim A request for payment of a loss indemnified by an insurance carrier.

Claimant An individual or an entity who makes an insurance claim.

Confidentiality The right of an individual to privacy.

Continued stay review A utilization review service that makes a request for approval of additional hospital inpatient days. This request is usually made by the hospital or attending physician. *Concurrent review* is another term used for this service.

Cost-benefit analysis A comparison and evaluation of costs and outcomes to maximize return on investment when choosing among medical alternatives. Cost-benefit analysis is used to determine the cost effectiveness of the case management plan and recommended services.

Cost containment Measures introduced to control or reduce the cost of medical care or other losses covered by insurance. May also refer to a philosophy of doing business that is directed at controlling costs.

Cost shifting The tendency to look for payment from other entities when the payment from the primary payer is inadequate to cover costs. Also, the practice of prorating financial losses from uninsured care among paying patients.

Coverage May refer to a line of insurance, such as life, workers' compensation, or medical, that pays benefits for certain types of risks. May also refer to the type and dollar limits of the benefits provided.

Covered lives All individuals who fall within the coverage of an insurance plan. This is different from subscribers, who are employees or others who actually subscribe to or pay for the coverage of a plan. Subscribers may have dependents (i.e., spouse or children) who are eligible for coverage.

Defendant The person or entity against whom a legal action is being brought.

Diagnosis-related groups (DRGs) Originally, this was a Medicare term that applied to a reimbursement system centered around flat-rate dollar amounts reimbursed on individual patients according to diagnoses, procedures, and other key factors (e.g., discharge status). In subsequent years, other insurance systems have adopted the concepts of this payment system.

Discharge planner An individual who coordinates services to ensure a client's timely and safe discharge from a facility or agency.

Disease management "A philosophy toward the treatment of the patient with an illness (usually chronic in nature) that seeks to prevent recurrence of symptoms, maintain high quality of life, and prevent future need for medical resources by using an integrated, comprehensive approach to health care. Pharmaceutical care, continuous quality improvement, practice guidelines, and case management all play key roles in this effort, which (in theory) will result in decreased health care costs as well."[137]

Durable medical equipment (DME) Medical apparatus, supplies, furniture, and so on that can be used over and over again for an extended period of time and is not considered to be consumable or disposable.

Employability statement A description by a qualified rehabilitation professional of an injured worker's ability to secure suitable gainful employment in light of the injured worker's education, training, experience, and physical capacities regardless of whether the injured worker has actually returned to work.

Employee Retirement Income Security Act of 1974 (ERISA) "A law that mandates reporting and disclosure requirements for group life and health plans."[138] This law governs self-funded health plans and is preempted by state law because of federal oversight.

Exclusion A medical condition, treatment, equipment, service, or other item that is not covered by an insurance plan.

Expert witness An individual who has special knowledge of a subject that is not possessed by the average person. Expert witnesses are called to testify in court on their special knowledge.

Fee-for-service This is a type of payment plan in which a specified monetary amount is reimbursed for delivery of a service. Fees-for-service can be fixed rates that cover a specified service or constellation of services aimed at a particular goal or outcome, or they can refer to an hourly rate.

Gainful employment Work that pays a wage.

Gatekeeper An individual who functions in the role of controlling access to services. Utilization review performs a gatekeeping function, as do primary care physicians/practitioners in HMOs.

Guardian ad litem A person appointed by a court to manage the affairs and safeguard the interests of a minor or an adult who has been judged incompetent to handle his or her own affairs.

Health maintenance organization (HMO) An organization that combines medical or health insurance with the provision of medical services through primary care practitioners and specified health care provider/facilities.

Home health care Medical services that are provided in the home to individuals who do not require hospitalization or nursing home care.

Hospice A health care system providing a constellation of services to persons who are terminally ill. Services may be provided at home or in a special live-in facility.

Indemnity Benefits paid by insurance companies for losses due to certain kinds of risks.

Independent medical examination (IME) A medical examination performed by another physician (not the attending physician) to obtain additional or corroborative information about a client's diagnosis, need for continued or additional treatment, degree of disability, and other factors.

Individualized vocational evaluation planning An organized process and set of techniques for developing and writing a plan to structure individual evaluations. It presupposes knowledge of the overall vocational evaluation process. Specific skills include planning and writing, as well as the ability to integrate information from clients and referral sources with other relevant data.

Initial assessment The assessment conducted by the case manager at the beginning of a case. This process may be conducted on-site or telephonically and usually involves conferring with the client/family, attending physician, and other individuals to determine the facts of the case so that case planning can take place.

Integrated delivery systems (IDS) Various health care delivery models involving strategic alliances among physicians, physician groups, hospitals, and other providers and practitioners.

Internet A worldwide network of computer networks that allows users to access information and communicate with one another all over the world.

Job analysis (JA) An in-depth description of a job that includes the duties, tasks, physical requirements, working conditions, and environmental conditions. A job analysis is often made by actually observing a worker performing a job.

Job modification Changes in a job that are made to accommodate a person with a disability. Job modifications can involve a change in duties and tasks or physical alterations in the work station or assistive devices.

Labor market survey (LMS) Employers are contacted in a systematic way to determine if work is available that a client can perform by virtue of skills, qualifications, and physical capacities.

Length of stay The number of days of inpatient hospitalization.

Liability insurance Insurance coverage designed to ensure against risks associated with causing harm to another through errors or omissions. Some of the most common forms of liability insurance include automobile, general or commercial, medical malpractice, and errors and omissions.

Long-term care Services that do not require inpatient hospitalization but must be provided under medical supervision for a lengthy period of time. This includes skilled nursing facilities, hospices, and intermediate care.

Long-term disability insurance (LTD) An income replacement insurance for people who become permanently or temporarily disabled. Medical benefits are not included in this type of coverage, but case management is sometimes used to assist in determining the extent of a claimant's disabilities, the ability to return to work, and the need for retraining.

Malingering Pretending to be ill or disabled.

Managed care "A system of healthcare delivery aimed at managing the cost and quality of access to healthcare. Managed care is used by HMOs, PPOs and managed indemnity plans to improve the delivery of services and contain costs."[139]

Maximum medical improvement (MMI) The point at which an individual achieves optimal recovery and maximum benefit from treatment. Sometimes called *maximum medical independence* or *medical stability.*

Medical reserving A process by which a claims adjuster estimates the amount of money necessary for the medical treatment of an injured worker. This may be based on the case manager's estimate of the severity of the condition and projected lengths and types of treatments/therapies necessary to achieve maximum medical improvement.

On-site case management This is provided through in-person visits and meetings by the case manager with the client/family, attending physician, hospital staff, employer, medical providers, and others to assess and coordinate care. Although in-person visits are made as necessary, much of the work also takes place telephonically and through other forms of communications.

Outcomes management A method of controlling medical costs through data analysis of outcomes of different treatment modalities for the same diagnosis. By collecting and analyzing this type of data, caregivers and third-party payers can obtain information on which modalities consistently result in better outcomes.

Panel examination A form of independent medical examination that involves the evaluation of an individual by a panel of physicians of different specialties. Often recommended as part of the process of settling an insurance claim, especially the determination of permanent disability.

Pension Permanent income replacement that is paid to workers' compensation recipients when they are permanently and totally disabled from working. Pensions usually replace income only partially.

Permanent partial disability (PPD) A disability that is not expected to improve sufficiently over time to permit an individual to engage in gainful employment without some restrictions. The individual may be able to engage in some jobs and some job activities but is restricted from others. PPD is often referred to as a lump sum award that is paid to an individual as part of an insurance settlement.

Permanent total disability (PTD) A disability that is not expected to improve sufficiently to permit an individual to engage in gainful employment. PTD is often referred to as an award (usually in the form of a pension) that is paid to an individual as part of an insurance settlement.

Physical capacities evaluation (PCE) One of several methods for determining what activities a person is capable of performing physically. The physical capacities usually evaluated include amount of weight that can be safely lifted or carried and tolerance for standing, sitting, walking, bending, crouching, crawling, climbing, kneeling, and so on. Sometimes, ability to tolerate certain environmental conditions (such as cold, heat, dust, fumes) is also evaluated. This type of evaluation can take place through simulations of these working conditions or through estimates by physicians who are familiar with objective medical findings.

Physician advisor A physician who acts as a consultant for a utilization review company or a case manager to assist in making determinations regarding the certification of services. Physician advisors are also used as resources in addressing the complex medical situations often encountered in case management.

Plaintiff A person who initiates a legal action based on the belief that an injury has occurred or rights have been violated.

Preferred provider organization (PPO) A third-party payer contracts with a group of medical professionals to provide services to its insured members at a discounted fee structure based on volume.

Prenotification/preauthorization certification Approval of an inpatient admission, outpatient procedure, or other medical service before implementation. Preadmission certification is a utilization review service. Often, a length of stay or service is assigned at the time of certification.

Primary care physician (PCP) The first physician a client sees, often referred to as a *family practitioner.* This physician screens clients for referral to a specialist or need for inpatient admission.

Quality assurance (QA) "the activity that monitors the level of care being provided by physicians, medical institutions, or any health care vendor in order to ensure that [patients] are receiving [appropriate care as] measured against preestablished standards, some of which are mandated by law."[140]

Quality of care Commonly accepted standards of care that indicate that a client has been provided adequate medical services given the nature of the diagnosis and other factors on the case.

Reinsurance carrier A type of insurance for insurance companies to counteract the adverse effects of large dollar claims. Sometimes referred to as *stop-loss insurance.*

Release to return to work A written authorization by an injured worker's attending physician allowing the injured worker to return to gainful employment, sometimes with certain physical restrictions.

Retrospective review A utilization review service that often takes place after service delivery. It is aimed at determining whether services provided were medically necessary and proper billing was done. Sometimes providers' practice patterns and hospital length of stay averages are also analyzed.

Second surgical opinion (SSO) The referral of a patient to another physician to determine the medical necessity of surgery that is being recommended by the attending physician. SSO is often requested on elective surgeries.

Sentinel effect An outcome of utilization review or managed care or other cost-containment procedures that reduces utilization or consumption of services.

Skilled nursing facility (SNF) Often referred to as a *nursing home,* this type of facility provides a high level of long-term care with 24-hour nursing care.

Standardized testing General knowledge of tests and measurements principles and the use of standardized instruments is employed to provide a quantitative assessment of an individual's cognitive, psychomotor, and affective traits. The required skills include selection, administration, modification, scoring, and interpretation, as well as a basic understanding of the theory of tests and measurements (i.e., validity, reliability, and norms).

Subscriber The individual who is employed by a company that has a group medical plan. May also be another individual who pays for or otherwise contracts for insurance coverage.

Suitable gainful employment (SGE) A job that is sufficiently remunerative in nature and is is considered to be substantive in nature. Some jurisdictions define SGE in terms of the individual's previous employment, education, and wage earning history.

Telephonic case management This type of case management takes place telephonically, by correspondence, and through electronic communications, such as e-mail, faxes, and modem transmissions. To save costs, it does not involve in-person visits.

Temporary partial disability (TPD) An indemnity payment made to a person to replace income when he or she is temporarily, partially unable to work due to a disability. This payment usually is made monthly and is often called "loss of earning power" on workers' compensation claims. TPD usually does not replace 100% of a person's income and is generally paid when the individual is only released for part-time work or work that pays less than the job at the time of injury.

Temporary total disability (TTD) An indemnity payment made to a person to replace income when he or she is temporarily unable to work due to a disability. This payment usually is made monthly and is often called "time-loss" on workers' compensation claims. TTD usually does not replace 100% of a person's income and is often capped.

Third-party administrator (TPA) A company that adjusts claims for another insurance company or an entity that is self-insured.

Time-loss Income replacement paid to workers' compensation claimants while they are temporarily unable to work. Sometimes called *indemnity.*

Transferrable skills Skills that are acquired through job experience, training, or education that may be used in more than one job and may qualify a worker for jobs that have not actually been performed as part of the work history.

Transitional return-to-work plan A temporary job modification that allows a worker who has been disabled to gradually adjust to returning to work. This may involve light-duty work, part-time work, or short shifts.

Utilization review (UR) A program implemented to control or limit (or both) the amount of health care services consumed by a member of a benefit plan. Some of the components of utilization review include preadmission certification, continued stay review, and retrospective review. The goal of utilization review is to reduce the number of unnecessary or inappropriate health care services while maintaining quality of care.

Vocational evaluation (VE) A systematic means for assessing clients' aptitudes, academic achievements, interests, dexterity, and temperaments as they apply to the world of work. This type of assessment usually includes the administration of standardized tests or work samples or both but may also involve job tryouts.

Vocational rehabilitation plan A written strategy for assisting a person with a vocational disability to become employable or obtain a job. Plans are usually written in a very specific, step-by-step manner that includes such services as job training, job placement, résumé development, and assistance with job-seeking skills.

Work hardening Simulation of a job that involves physical capacities related to those required on the actual job. An individual performs this simulation over a period of time to develop the physical conditioning required to perform the job.

Work history The jobs, education, training, and skills acquired through hobbies or avocations that make up a person's background as it relates to the world of work.

Workers' compensation A type of insurance that covers injuries and illnesses that are job related. Workers' compensation is a no-fault system (in nearly all jurisdictions) whereby the worker gives up the right to sue the employer in exchange for the payment of medical and time-loss benefits.

SUGGESTED READINGS

Medicom International: *Managed care A thru Z, managed care terms,* Bronxville, NY, 1996, Author.

Mullahy CM: *The case manager's handbook,* Gaithersburg, Md, 1995, Aspen.

Rehabilitation Committee of the Southern Association of Workmen's Compensation Administrators: The workers' compensation rehabilitation process: definitions, standards, and procedures, *NARPPS J News* 6(5):195-198, 1991.

References are found at the end of the book.

REFERENCES

1. Lewin SS, Ramseur JH, Sink JM: The role of private rehabilitation: founder, catalyst, competitor, *J Rehabil* 45(3):16-19, 1979.
2. Siefker JM: What is the difference between public and private sector rehabilitation? In Siefker JM, editor: *Vocational evaluation in private sector rehabilitation,* Menomonie, Wisc, 1992, The Rehabilitation Resource, University of Wisconsin-Stout.
3. Gerson V: George T. Welch: the father of modern case management, *Case Manager,* pp 71-75, Sept-Oct 1996.
4. Boling J: Foreword. In Mullahy CM: *The case manager's handbook,* Gaithersburg, Md, 1995, Aspen, p ix.
5. Merrill JC: Defining case management, *Business and Health* 3:5-9, 1985.
6. Abramowski D and others: NARPPS professional performance criteria for medical case management, *NARPPS J News* 5(6): 111-115, 1990.
7. Commission for Case Manager Certification: *CCM certification guide, certified case manager,* Rolling Meadows, Ill, 1996, Author.
8. Case Management Society of America: *CMSA, Case Management Society of America, standards of practice,* Little Rock, Ark, 1995, Author, p 8.
9. Mullahy CM: *The case manager's handbook,* Gaithersburg, Md, 1995, Aspen.
10. Cohen EL, Cesta TG: *Nursing case management: from concept to evaluation,* ed 2, St. Louis, 1997, Mosby.
11. Commission for Case Manager Certification: *CCM certification guide, certified case manager,* Rolling Meadows, Ill, 1996, Author.
12. Smith DS: Standards of practice for case management: the importance of practice standards, *J Care Management* 1(3):6, 1995.
13. Ibid, p 5.
14. Gerson V: George T. Welch: the father of modern case management, *Case Manager,* pp 71-75, Sept-Oct 1996.
15. Case Management Society of America: *CMSA, Case Management Society of America, standards of practice,* Little Rock, Ark, 1995, Author.
16. Commission for Case Manager Certification: *CCM certification guide, certified case manager,* Rolling Meadows, Ill, 1996, Author.
17. Ibid, p 4.
18. Ibid, p 5.
19. Case Management Society of America: *CMSA, Case Management Society of America, standards of practice,* Little Rock, Ark, 1995, Author, pp 18-19.
20. Ibid, pp 18-19.
21. Abramowski D and others: NARPPS professional performance criteria for medical case management, *NARPPS J News* 5(6): 111-115, 1990.
22. Romaine DS: Case management challenges, present and future, *Continuing Care* 14(1):24-31, 1995.
23. Choppa AJ and others: Vocational rehabilitation counselors as case managers, *Case Manager,* pp 45-50, Sept-Oct 1996.
24. Specialized CM raises professional credibility, *Case Management Advisor* 5(8):108-112, 1994.
25. Ibid.
26. Romaine DS: Case management challenges, present and future, *Continuing Care* 14(1):24-31, 1995.

27. Ernst & Young: *Hospital-physician integration: results of a national survey,* Washington, DC, June 1993, Author.
28. Mullahy CM: *The case manager's handbook,* Gaithersburg, Md, 1995, Aspen, p 5.
29. Will new Medicaid CM regs lead to documentation overhaul for states? *Case Management Advisor* 5(3):29, 1994.
30. Gann C, Moreland T: Introduction to insurance and workers' compensation. In Siefker JM, editor: *Vocational evaluation in private sector rehabilitation,* Menomonie, Wisc, 1992, The Rehabilitation Resource.
31. Ibid, p 71.
32. Study finds CMs return employees to work faster, *Case Management Advisor* 6(8):113-114, 1995.
33. Choppa A and others: Life care planning and mediation, *Rehabil Rev* 2(5):3-5, 1994.
34. Hogue EE: Are case managers liable? *J Care Management* 1(2):35-38,53, 1995.
35. Romaine DS: Case management challenges, present and future, *Continuing Care* 14(1):24-31, 1995.
36. Coleman JR: New challenges call for rewriting the rules for problem solving, *Case Manager* 7(2):47-50, 1996.
37. Mullahy CM: *The case manager's handbook,* Gaithersburg, Md, 1995, Aspen, pp 161-169.
38. New York, 1979, Macmillan.
39. American Psychiatric Association, Washington, DC, 1994, Author.
40. American Psychiatric Association: *Diagnostic and statistical manual of mental disorders—IV,* Washington, DC, 1994, Author, p 25.
41. Ibid, p 25.
42. Ibid, pp 29-30.
43. Ibid, p 32.
44. Taking your case (management) to court, *Case Management Advisor* 5(5):73-74, 1995.
45. Dress for success as expert witness, *Case Management Advisor* 5(4):58-59, 1995.
46. Find, persuade key buyers of CM services; here's how, *Case Management Advisor* 6(4): 54-56, 1995.
47. Garrett MB: Selling and marketing a case management program, *Case Manager* 6(4): 59-66, 1995.
48. Get involved early to reduce clients' workers' comp costs, speed return to work, *Case Management Advisor* 5(12):161-164, 1994.
49. Software takes big byte out of CM workload, *Case Management Advisor* 6(7):93-94, 99-101, 1995.
50. Maehling JA, Badger K: Information systems tools available to the case manager, *Nursing Case Management* 1(1):35-40, 1996.
51. Computerization: don't byte off more bits than you can chew, *Case Management Advisor* 6(2):17-21, 1995.
52. Van Genderen A: How to develop and manage a case management department, *J Care Management* 2(4):30-41, 1996.
53. Computerization: don't byte off more bits than you can chew, *Case Management Advisor* 6(2):17-21, 1995.
54. Lowery SL: Hiring right—Qualifications for the successful case manager, *Case Manager* 3(4):66-68, 70-71, 73-74, 1992.
55. Ibid.
56. Gaithersburg, Md, 1995, Aspen.
57. Meeks K and others: Guidelines for supervision of medical case management, *NARPPS J News* 6(6):251-255, 1991.
58. Case management caseloads: how much is too much? *Case Management Advisor* 6(5): 61-64, 1995.
59. Clear, complete communication helps CMs safely navigate legal minefields, *Case Management Advisor* 8(3):41-44, 1997.
60. Case Management Society of America: *CMSA, Case Management Society of America, standards of practice,* Little Rock, Ark, 1995, Author.
61. Hogue EE: Are case managers liable? *J Care Management* 1(2):35-38, 1995.
62. Geron SM, Chassler D: *Guidelines for case management practice across the long-term care continuum,* Boston, 1994, Boston University School of Social Work, p 72.
63. Meeks K and others: Guidelines for supervision of medical case management, *NARPPS J News* 6(6):251-255, 1991.

64. Gaucher EJ, Coffey RJ: *Total quality in healthcare,* San Francisco, 1993, Jossey-Bass, p 57.
65. Are members getting CM satisfaction? *Case Management Advisor* 6(9):118, 1995.
66. Ibid.
67. Romaine DS: Outcomes measurements—tools for case management decisions, *Continuing Care* 14(2):34-38, 1995.
68. Healy BM: Early intervention, physical therapy and industrial rehabilitation: prescription for success, *Continuing Care* 14(2):15-18, 1995.
69. No yardstick for measuring CM outcomes yet—but change is on the way, *Case Management Advisor* 5(4):133-137, 1994.
70. A brief look at rehab outcomes measures for case managers, *Case Management Advisor* 5(4):49-51, 1994.
71. Outcomes measurement tools can boost your CM efforts, ensure better patient oversight, *Case Management Advisor* 5(4):46-49, 1994.
72. Understanding outcomes data to make informed CM decisions, *Case Management Advisor* 5(6):77-79, 1995.
73. The workers' compensation rehabilitation process: definitions, standards, and procedures, *NARPPS J News* 6(5):195-198, 1991.
74. Cassidy J: A hard look at work hardening programs: selecting a provider in this expanding industry calls for a thorough approach, *Continuing Care* 12(2):22-26, 1993.
75. Rubin SE, Roessler RT: *Foundations of the vocational rehabilitation process,* ed 2, Austin, Tex, 1983, Pro-ed, pp 113-114.
76. US Department of Labor: Washington, DC, 1991, US Government Printing Office.
77. Field TF, Field JF: *Classification of jobs,* Athens, Ga, 1992, Elliott & Fitzpatrick.
78. Havranek J and others: Athens, Ga, 1994, Elliott & Fitzpatrick.
79. Cutler F, Ramm A: Introduction to the basics of vocational evaluation. In Siefker JM, editor: *Vocational evaluation in private sector rehabilitation,* Menomonie, Wisc, 1992, The Rehabilitation Resource.
80. Ibid.
81. Pyle DW: *Intelligence: an introduction,* London, 1979, Routledge & Kegan Paul.
82. Siefker JM: *Tests and test use in vocational evaluation and assessment,* Menomonie, Wisc, 1996, The Rehabilitation Resource.
83. Cutler F, Ramm A: Introduction to the basics of vocational evaluation. In Siefker JM, editor: *Vocational evaluation in private sector rehabilitation,* Menomonie, Wisc, 1992, The Rehabilitation Resource.
84. Ibid.
85. National Council on Disability: *Americans with Disabilities Act signed by President Bush, July 26, 1990,* Washington, DC, Author, p 4.
86. Walker JM: The Americans with Disabilities Act and the rehabilitation CM, *Case Manager* 3(3):41-42, 44, 46, 1992.
87. Gibson K, Jayne K: Reasonable accommodation: a cornerstone of ADA compliance for employers, *NARPPS J News* 7(4):139-142, 1992.
88. Case Management Society of America: CMSA statement regarding ethical case management practice, *J Care Management* 2(2):8-9, 1996.
89. CMSA: *Standards of practice,* Little Rock, Ark, 1995, Author.
90. Abramowski D and others: NARPPS professional performance criteria for medical case management, *NARPPS J News* 5(6): 111-115, 1990.
91. Rodwin MA: Conflicts in managed care, *N Engl J Med* 332(9):604-607, 1995.
92. Boling J: Profile: John Banja, *Case Manager* 2(3):76, 78-79, 1991.
93. CMSA: Proposed CMSA statement regarding ethical case management practice, *J Care Management* 1(1):33, 1995.
94. CMSA: *Standards of practice,* Little Rock, Ark, 1995, Author, p 20.
95. Siefker JM: What is the difference between public and private sector rehabilitation? In Siefker JM, editor: *Vocational evaluation in private sector rehabilitation,* Menomonie, Wisc, 1992, The Rehabilitation Resource, pp 1-29.
96. Banja JD: Ethics: conflicts of interest: I, *Case Manager* 2(4):24, 26, 1991.

97. Banja JD: Ethics: conflicts of interest: II, *Case Manager* 3(1):20, 22, 1991.
98. McClinton DH: Balancing the issue of ethics in case management, *Continuing Care* 14(5):13-16, 1995.
99. Ibid.
100. Banja JD: Ethics: if momma dies, you die, *Case Manager* 7(1):37-40, 1996.
101. American Health Consultants: Giving disabled "right to risk" speeds rehab, *Case Management Advisor* 6(5):66, 71-73, 1995.
102. Banja JD: Ethics: when we have to pay for someone else's risk taking, *Case Manager* 7(21):32-34, 1996.
103. McClinton DH: Balancing the issue of ethics in case management, *Continuing Care* 14(5):13-14, 16, 1995.
104. American Health Consultants: Use disease state management to reduce costs through prevention, *Case Management Advisor* 6(8): 105-107, 1995.
105. Disease management faces obstacle, *Modern Healthcare,* pp 30-33, 1995.
106. Ward MD, Rieve J: Disease management: case management's return to patient-centered care, *J Care Management* 1(4):7-12, 1995.
107. Eichert JH: *Systems-based disease management,* Paper presented at Medical Case Management Convention VIII, Orlando, Fla, 1996.
108. Zitter M: *Special report: disease management,* San Francisco, 1994, The Zitter Group.
109. Eichert JH: *Systems-based disease management,* Paper presented at Medical Case Management Convention VIII, Orlando, Fla, 1996.
110. American Health Consultants: Use disease state management to reduce costs through prevention, *Case Management Advisor* 6(8): 105-107, 1995.
111. American Health Consultants: HMO: disease state management is essential, *Case Management Advisor* 6(9):129-131, 1995.
112. Ward MD, Rieve J: Disease management: case management's return to patient-centered care, *J Care Management* 1(4):7-12, 1995.
113. Tanouye L: *Riding the waves of culture shock thru rehabilitation counseling,* Paper presented at the WA NARPPS Spring Conference, June 20, 1996.
114. American Health Consultants: Changes in US demographics force CMs to address patients' cultural diversity, *Case Management Advisor* 5(11):145-150, 1994.
115. Leal-Idrogo A: Further thoughts on the use of interpreters and translators in delivery of rehabilitation services, *J Rehabil* 61(2): 21-23, 1995.
116. American Health Consultants: Changes in US demographics force CMs to address patients' cultural diversity, *Case Management Advisor* 5(11):145-150, 1994.
117. Feist-Price S, Ford-Harris D: Rehabilitation counseling: issues specific to providing services to African American clients, *J Rehabil* 60(4):13-19, 1994.
118. Ibid.
119. Ibid.
120. Rogers C: *On becoming a person,* Boston, 1961, Houghton Mifflin.
121. Chrisman N: Culture-sensitive healthcare, Sixth Annual Northwest Medical Case Management Conference, Seattle, 1995, Author, p 1.
122. American Health Consultants: Changes in U.S. demographics force CMs to address patients' cultural diversity, *Case Management Advisor* 5(11):145-150, 1994.
123. Ibid, p 3.
124. Kleinman A, Eisenberg L, Good B: Culture, illness, and care: clinical lessons from anthropologic and cross-cultural research, *Ann Intern Med* 88:251-258, 1978.
125. Get involved early to reduce clients' workers' comp costs, speed return to work, *Case Management Advisor* 5(12):161-164, 1994.
126. Mullahy CM: Case managers and physicians: working associates, not adversaries, *Case Manager* 3(2):62-68, 1992.
127. Reich P: Capitation and ethics, *Med Interface* 9(9):16, 1996.
128. Council on Ethical and Judicial Affairs: Ethical issues in managed care, *JAMA* 273(4):330-335, 1995.

129. Gries L, Jorgensen C, McNeely E: Case management in a school of nursing: a cooperative effort, *Case Manager* 2(4):30, 32, 34, 36, 38, 1991.
130. Choppa A and others: Life care planning and mediation, *Rehabil Rev* 2(5):3-5, 1994.
131. *Dictionary of occupational titles: fourth edition, revised 1991*, Washington, DC, 1991, US Department of Labor, p xv.
132. Maze M, Mayall D, Farr JM: *Enhanced guide for occupational exploration*, ed 2 rev, Indianapolis, 1995, JIST-Works.
133. *Dictionary of occupational titles: fourth edition, revised 1991*, Washington, DC, 1991, US Department of Labor, p xiii.
134. Field T, Field J: *Classification of jobs*, Athens, Ga, 1992, Elliott & Fitzpatrick.
135. Maze M, Mayall D, Farr JM: *Enhanced guide for occupational exploration*, ed 2 rev, Indianapolis, 1995, JIST-Works.
136. Medicom International: *Managed care A thru Z, managed care terms*, Bronxville, NY, 1996, Author, p 4.
137. Ibid, p 22.
138. Ibid, p 25.
139. Mullahy CM: *The case manager's handbook*, Gaithersburg, Md, 1995, Aspen, p 390.
140. Medicom International: *Managed care A thru Z, managed care terms*, Bronxville, NY, 1996, Author, p 56.

INDEX